Decoding Medical Careers: A Teenage Guide to Medical Specialties

Aleeza Raza

Introduction

In the world of medicine, every heartbeat, breath, and diagnosis presents an opportunity to change someone's life. *Decoding Medical Careers: A Teenage Guide to Medical Specialties* navigates 20 medical specialties with descriptions, fun facts, trivia, and interviews with medical professionals! From the adrenaline-filled emergency room to the operating room, each specialty has its own charm and provides a tremendous amount of patient care. In the quest to decode medical specialties, fascinating facts about each career are shared. Did you know that dermatologists can diagnose certain conditions just by examining your nails? Did you know that radiologists can decipher medical images like puzzle pieces? This book provides insightful interviews with doctors who have dedicated their careers to care for others. Discover their stories, challenges, and knowledge. Their personal experiences guide readers as they navigate their journey toward medicine. Trivia questions are sprinkled throughout the pages of this book to test readers on their medical knowledge. Did you know that the longest surgery on record lasted longer than four days? Readers will be educated as they discover small pieces of medical information. This book not only highlights various medical specialties but outlines the journey and steps to becoming each type of physician. Each type of physician goes through years of schooling and training, and each step of their journey is explained thoroughly. Tailored for teenagers, it empowers them with the knowledge to navigate the intricate path to a fulfilling medical career. *Decoding Medical Careers: A Teenage Guide to Medical Specialties* is a compass to help readers navigate the vast ocean of medical possibilities. If you dream of becoming a pediatrician, who heals the youngest of patients, or an anesthesiologist who ensures pain-free surgeries, this guide equips readers with all the knowledge and inspiration needed to make informed decisions about careers in medicine. Let the decoding begin!

Decoding Medical Careers: A Teenage Guide to Medical Specialties

Table of Contents

Anesthesiology……………………………………………………………….. 4

Cardiology……………………………….. ……………………………… 10

Dermatology………………………………………………………………. 16

Emergency Medicine……………………………………………………. 22

Family Medicine………………………………………………………….. 28

Gastroenterology…………………………………………………………. 34

General Surgery………………………………………………………….. 40

Internal Medicine…………………………………………………………. 46

Nephrology……………………………………………………………….. 52

Neurology & Neurosurgery…………………………………………….. 58

Obstetrics & Gynecology………………………………………………. 64

Oncology………………………………………………………………….. 70

Optometry & Ophthalmology…………………………………………. 76

Orthopedics………………………………………………………………82

Pathology…………………………………………………………………. 88

Pediatrics…………………………………………………………………. 94

Plastic Surgery…………………………………………………………. 100

Psychiatry……………………………………………………………….. 106

Radiology……………………………………………………………….. 112

Urology………………………………………………………………….. 118

Interviews………………………………………………………………..123

Author's note…………………………………………………………… 127

Anesthesiology

An anesthesiologist is a doctor who practices anesthesia. They specialize in perioperative care (before, during, and after surgery), they develop anesthetic plans for their patients, and administer anesthetics. An anesthesiologist's role extends far beyond administering medication to induce unconsciousness during surgery. They meet with their patient and the surgeon to discuss anesthetic care so it is safe and effective. They will discuss their patient's overall health, medical history, and address any questions or concerns. A preoperative (before surgery) evaluation is necessary in determining the most appropriate anesthesia technique, and to minimize any potential complications. They tailor anesthesia plans for each individual patient considering their medical history, surgical procedure, age, and potential risks. There are several types of anesthesia. General anesthesia is when the patient is unconscious and has no awareness. Regional anesthesia numbs a specific area of the body to prevent the patient from feeling any pain. Sedation is when medications are given via IV to make a patient feel soothed and drowsy. During surgery, an anesthesiologist will monitor their patients' anesthesia and vital body functions. They are in control of their patient's pain level and their unconsciousness during an operation. Anesthesiologists are responsible for ensuring the patient's safety and making immediate adjustments if any issues or complications arise. They are trained to respond quickly and effectively to emergencies that may occur during surgery, such as reactions to anesthesia, cardiac events, or respiratory problems. Their expertise in resuscitation and critical care is essential in these situations. When surgery is complete, the anesthesiologist will begin to slowly wake the patient. The term for waking up from anesthesia is called emergence. Anesthesiologists will take care of their patients after surgery to make sure they are comfortable and not in any pain. They can administer pain-relief medications and design post-operative pain management plans to ensure that their patients are as comfortable as possible during the recovery process. Anesthesiologists make sure that their patients wake up safely and are stable before transferring them to the Post-Anesthesia Care Unit (PACU). Anesthesiologists also provide anesthesia services for many medical procedures outside of surgery, such as childbirth. They work closely with surgical teams, nurses, and other medical professionals to ensure the safety and comfort of their patients. Overall, anesthesiologists are vital medical professionals inside and out of the operating room and ensure that patients receive safe and effective anesthesia.

The road to becoming an anesthesiologist is challenging and rigorous. The first step on this road begins with completing a bachelor's degree, typically in a science-related field. Students must take the MCAT (Medical College Admissions Test) for acceptance into medical school. Taking the MCAT requires months of preparation. Following the completion of their undergraduate studies, they undertake the challenge of gaining acceptance into medical school. An excellent medical school application includes volunteer hours, clinical experience, a high GPA, a competitive MCAT score, and strong recommendation letters. During their medical school training, they learn to decipher complex medical cases, develop critical thinking skills, and dive into the vast sea of medical knowledge. They also learn core subjects such as pharmacology, biochemistry, anatomy, and medical ethics. In the final years of medical school, students must decide which specialty they are most interested in, and apply for residency. Anesthesia residency is 4 years long. Residency allows aspiring anesthesiologists to work with experienced physicians, assess patients, and gain experience in the operating room. The period of residency demands long hours and large responsibilities. Throughout the years of medical school and residency, physicians must complete all steps of the USMLE (United States Medical Licensing Exam) or COMLEX (Comprehensive Osteopathic Medical Licensing Exam). There are three steps of these exams, the first two parts are typically taken during medical school. Next, they have the option of completing a fellowship. A fellowship in anesthesia provides additional training in subspecialties such as cardiac anesthesia, pediatric anesthesia, neuroanesthesia, and more. Anesthesiology fellowships are typically 1-year in length. Anesthesiologists can become board-certified once they take and pass an exam by the American Board of Anesthesia. Board certification is not required, but it demonstrates a physician's competency in their field. Next, in order to begin practicing medicine in their location, they must obtain a license. Every medical specialty is constantly evolving, so their learning is not yet complete. They must regularly complete continuing education courses to stay up to date on best practices in patient care. The road to becoming an anesthesiologist demands sacrifice, perseverance, and commitment. The anesthesiologists who successfully navigated this road have the opportunity to make an impact on their patients' lives and to provide them with expert care.

Why You Should Become an Anesthesiologist

One of the Highest-paying medical careers

The average anesthesiologist makes $350,000+ a year

Work Variety

They may administer anesthesia to a delivering mother, a child receiving a life-saving surgery, or an elderly patient having a routine procedure

Work-Life Balance

50% of anesthesiologists claim they can take a 4-week vacation annually

Exhilaration

Anesthesiologists are in control of their patient's consciousness and are responsible for waking them up.

Decoding Medical Careers: A Teenage Guide to Medical Specialties

Anesthesia Trivia

1. What does regional anesthesia do?

    a. Makes the patient unconscious and completely unaware

    b. Makes the patient drowsy and relaxed

    c. Numbs a specific area of the patient's body

    d. Results in irreversible numbness of a limb

2. Another term for Nitrous Oxide is ____

    a. Laughing gas

    b. Crying gas

    c. Tear gas

    d. Numbing gel

3. A typical Anesthesia residency lasts how many years?

    a. 6 years

    b. 4 years

    c. 2 years

    d. 3 years

4. What portion of the nerve do local anesthetics work on?

    a. Neurons

    b. Nerve membrane

    c. Dendrites

    d. Nerve clusters

All answers on next page

Anesthesia Trivia

1. What does regional anesthesia do?

    a. Makes the patient unconscious and completely unaware

    b. Makes the patient drowsy and relaxed

    c. Numbs a specific area of the patient's body

    d. Results in irreversible numbness of a limb

2. Another term for Nitrous Oxide is ___

    a. Laughing gas

    b. Crying gas

    c. Tear gas

    d. Numbing gel

3. A typical anesthesia residency lasts how many years?

    a. 6 years

    b. 4 years

    c. 2 years

    d. 3 years

4. What portion of the nerve do local anesthetics work on?

    a. Neurons

    b. Nerve membrane

    c. Dendrites

    d. Nerve clusters

Anesthesia Fun Facts

1. People who smoke may need more anesthesia than nonsmokers

2. Anesthesiologists are currently ranked as the Number #1 best-paying job

3. Being overweight can increase the risk of anesthetic complications

4. The word "anesthesia" comes from the Greek language and means "loss of sensation" or "lack of sense of touch"

5. General anesthesia is the most common form of anesthesia

6. Anesthesia was first publicly demonstrated on October 16th, 1846 by William T.G Morton

Cardiology

Cardiology is the branch of medicine that focuses on preventing, treating, and diagnosing heart conditions. Cardiologists are dedicated to understanding the intricacies of the heart's function, structure, and various conditions that can affect the human body's health. They may work in hospitals or in private practices. The heart pumps oxygenated blood through blood vessels and throughout the rest of the body, making it the most important organ of the circulatory system. Cardiologists can treat heart failure, chest pain, and high blood pressure. They can order tests like electrocardiograms and echocardiograms which record the electrical activity of the heart. A commonly used tool in cardiology is a stress test, which monitors a patient's heart rhythm and blood pressure while they run or walk on a treadmill, or ride a bike. Cardiologists may use imaging techniques such as MRIs and CT scans to obtain detailed images of the heart. Once a heart condition is diagnosed, treatment options may include medications, lifestyle modifications, or in some cases surgery. A cardiac surgeon specializes in surgery of the heart and its major blood vessels. A cardiothoracic surgeon performs surgery on anything inside the chest, such as your heart, lungs, and esophagus. They can perform heart transplants, treat heart failure and issues with the aorta. The aorta is the largest artery in the body, it carries blood from the heart throughout the rest of the body. Pediatric or congenital heart surgeons are highly specialized professionals who focus on the surgical treatment of heart conditions in children, infants, and adults. They perform complex surgeries often on young patients who have congenital heart abnormalities that are usually present from birth. They repair heart defects such as a hole in the heart, heart valve defects, and atresia. Atresia is when a valve is not formed correctly, or has no opening to let blood pass through. The heart is an intricate structure, it includes several ventricles, arteries, and veins. Cardiologists, cardiac surgeons, cardiothoracic surgeons, and congenital heart surgeons deeply understand the complexity of the heart. The collaboration between these medical professionals has significantly contributed to the progress made in treating cardiovascular diseases. The field of cardiology places importance on preventative care. They educate patients about risk factors such as high blood pressure, high cholesterol and encourage regular physical activity to maintain heart health. Overall, cardiology is a dynamic specialty that focuses on the well-being of the heart and the circulatory system. Cardiologists hope to improve the lives of individuals affected by cardiovascular diseases and ailments.

Becoming a cardiologist requires a significant amount of commitment toward education and training. First, obtain a bachelor's degree, in a science-related field. It is important to maintain a high GPA (Grade Point Average), and to take the prerequisite courses for medical school. These courses include physics, chemistry, biology, organic chemistry, biochemistry, and more. It is required to take the MCAT (Medical College Admissions Test) in order to attend medical school. Once accepted into medical school, you will need to obtain an M.D. (Doctor of Medicine) or D.O. (Doctor of Osteopathic Medicine) degree. The difference between the two is that MDs typically take a more medication-focused approach to medicine, while DOs take a more holistic approach to medicine. Medical school typically takes 4 years. The first two years of medical school consist of classroom-based learning on subjects such as biochemistry, anatomy, pharmacology, and more. The last two years of medical school consist of clinical rotations in several medical specialties, including cardiology. These clinical rotations are graded, and high rotation grades are crucial for residency. Prospective cardiologists must then complete a residency program in internal medicine, which takes 3 years. During this time residents gain experience treating and diagnosing medical conditions, including cardiovascular diseases. An internal medicine residency is the foundation for further specialization in the field of cardiology. Throughout the 7 years of medical school and residency, physicians must complete all three steps of the USMLE (United States Medical Licensing Exam) or COMLEX (Comprehensive Osteopathic Medical Licensing Exam). Following the completion of an internal medicine residency, aspiring cardiologists must apply for a fellowship in cardiology. During the fellowship, they have the opportunity to work alongside experienced cardiologists and gain hands-on exposure to cardiologic procedures. This period is much more advanced and is extremely in-depth. After completing all of their training cardiologists can take an exam by the ABIM (American Board of Internal Medicine) or the AOBIM (American Osteopathic Board of Internal Medicine) to become board-certified. They must pass either of these exams to become a board-certified cardiologist. Most of the questions on the exams are realistic patient scenarios and identification skills. It tests their knowledge, skills, and competency in the field of cardiology. Cardiology offers several subspecialties such as pediatric cardiology, interventional cardiology, and advanced heart failure and transplant cardiology. If you choose to specialize further, you can pursue additional fellowships in these subspecialties. It takes a minimum of 10 years to become a cardiologist, but it is an especially rewarding field.

Why You Should Become a Cardiologist

Saving Lives

Cardiologists deal with matters between life and death throughout their careers. They have a direct impact on their patients by treating one of the most important organs in the human body.

Not Just Surgery

There is variety in cardiology, and there are many roles that do not always require surgery. You may perform tests and use other non-invasive methods to treat patients.

Respected Profession

Cardiologists are experts in their field.

High Salary

The average cardiologist in the U.S. makes $405,000+ a year

Decoding Medical Careers: A Teenage Guide to Medical Specialties

Cardiology Trivia

1. How many chambers does the heart have?
    a. 4
    b. 3
    c. 2
    d. 5

2. Men and women have different heart attack symptoms.
    a. True
    b. False

3. What is the largest artery in the human body?
    a. The right coronary artery
    b. Left coronary artery
    c. The aorta
    d. Circumflex artery

4. Around how many times does the heart beat every day?
    a. Around 150,000 times a day
    b. Around 100,000 times a day
    c. Around 76,000 times a day
    d. Around 62,000 times a day

All answers on next page

Cardiology Trivia

1. How many chambers does the heart have?
    a. 4
    b. 3
    c. 2
    d. 5

2. Men and women have different heart attack symptoms.
    a. True
    b. False

3. What is the largest artery in the human body?
    a. The right coronary artery
    a. Left coronary artery
    b. The aorta
    c. Circumflex artery

4. Around how many times does the heart beat every day?
    a. Around 160,000 times a day
    b. Around 100,000 times a day
    c. Around 76,000 times a day
    d. Around 62,000 times a day

Decoding Medical Careers: A Teenage Guide to Medical Specialties

Cardio Fun Facts

1. Your heart pumps 2,000 gallons of blood a day

2. The aorta is an inch in diameter, it is like a garden hose

3. There are 60,000 miles of blood vessels in the body

4. Heart disease is the #1 cause of death in the United States

5. Most heart attacks happen on a Monday

6. Whales have the largest hearts of any mammals

7. The youngest person to receive heart surgery was only a minute old

Dermatology

The skin is the human body's largest organ, it provides clues about your overall health, and a dermatologist specializes in its care. Dermatology is a specialized medical field that focuses on the diagnosis, treatment, and prevention of conditions related to the hair, skin, and nails. Dermatology encompasses a wide range of conditions, from common skin issues like acne and eczema to more serious conditions like skin cancer. Dermatologists are trained medical professionals who provide comprehensive care for patients with dermatological concerns. They may change the life of a young woman struggling with hair loss, treat an elderly woman's skin cancer at an early stage, or treat the acne of an insecure teenager. By looking at your skin or nails they may be able to identify symptoms that hint towards internal conditions or vitamin deficiencies. Dermatologists possess a great understanding of the anatomy and physiology of the skin which allows them to identify many skin diseases and disorders. Through careful examination, medical history evaluations, and tests, a dermatologist can determine the nature and severity of a condition. They can diagnose and properly treat over 3,000 diseases of the hair, skin, and nails. Once a diagnosis is made, dermatologists use their expertise to recommend and prescribe treatments. They may prescribe topical or oral medications, perform dermatologic procedures, or advise patients with lifestyle changes. Dermatologists can perform various dermatological procedures such as mole removal, laser surgery, and Mohs surgery. Mohs surgery is a procedure that is used to treat skin cancer lesions. They also help patients with cosmetic concerns, like wrinkles, sagging skin, and discoloration. Dermatologists may specialize in subspecialty fields such as pediatric dermatology, Mohs surgery, cosmetic dermatology, and more. Cosmetic procedures they can perform are botox injections, dermal fillers, and skin tightening. These procedures enhance the appearance of the skin and improve a patient's self-confidence. Preventative care is a crucial aspect of dermatology. Dermatologists educate their patients about sun protection and the early detection of skin cancer. By promoting awareness and early detection, dermatologists reduce the impact of life-threatening skin diseases. Dermatologists recommend getting skin cancer screenings once a year, and to apply sunscreen every day. In conclusion, dermatology is a diverse medical field concerned with the health of the hair, skin, and nails. By combining surgical skills and medical knowledge, dermatologists play a significant role in promoting skin health and improving their patient's well-being.

Becoming a dermatologist requires specialized training and dedication. It begins with obtaining a bachelor's degree typically in a science-related field, such as biology or chemistry. It's important to fulfill the prerequisite courses for medical school. The next step requires getting accepted and attending medical school. Acceptance into medical school requires a high GPA, a satisfactory score on the MCAT (Medical College Admissions Test), and excellent letters of recommendation. Medical school typically takes 4 years to complete. Following medical school, aspiring dermatologists must complete one year of an internship. After their internship, aspiring dermatologists must complete a residency program in dermatology. This includes hands-on clinical experience, research opportunities, and working under the guidance of experienced dermatologists. Dermatology residencies last three to four years. It's important to remember that dermatology is a highly competitive field, and is difficult to match into. The first reason is because the number of students who apply is greater than the number of spots available. The second reason is that dermatology is in the top five specialties for physician happiness and compensation. Having good board scores, rotation grades, letters of recommendation, and research can increase your chances of being accepted into a dermatology residency program. After their residency, future dermatologists have the option to complete a fellowship. A fellowship will offer additional training in a dermatological subspecialty. Subspecialties within dermatology include pediatric dermatology, Mohs surgery, dermatologic surgery, and more. To begin practicing medicine in their location a dermatologist must obtain a license. Dermatologists also have the option to become board-certified, this involves passing a lengthy exam issued by the American Board of Dermatology. This is an exam that will test their knowledge and competency in the field of dermatology. Even after becoming a well-established dermatologist, it is important to note that dermatology is a rapidly evolving field. It is essential for dermatologists to stay updated on the new techniques and research within their specialty. This involves participating in medical education activities, attending conferences, and more. Becoming a dermatologist requires dedication and a genuine passion for dermatology. It is a unique career that allows physicians to make a positive impact on their patient's lives by addressing their dermatological needs.

Why You Should Become a Dermatologist

Fulfilling Speciality

Dermatology is highly fulfilling because there is so much variety, everyone's skin is different

Excellent Work-Life Balance

They work a predictable schedule with regular hours, they aren't many "dermatologic emergencies"

Job Satisfaction

Dermatologists can possibly save multiple lives every day. They remove one melanoma, and they can save someone's life. They directly impact their patients.

In Demand

Dermatologists are currently in demand

Decoding Medical Careers: A Teenage Guide to Medical Specialties

Dermatology Trivia

1. The skin renews itself every ____
    a. 7 years
    b. 3 years
    c. 14 days
    d. 28 days

2. The average person has how many skin cells?
    a. 300 million
    b. 100 million
    c. 450 million
    d. 230 million

3. The skin is composed of how many primary layers?
    a. 6
    b. 3
    c. 4
    d. 9

4. What is Rosacea?
    a. A skin condition that causes blushing or visible blood vessels on the face
    b. When the immune system attacks the cells in the epidermis and the mucous membranes
    c. Patchy hair loss
    d. A condition that causes the skin to be dry, flaky, and bumpy

All answers on next page

Dermatology Trivia

1. The skin renews itself every ____
    a. 7 years
    b. 3 years
    c. 14 days
    d. 28 days

2. The average person has how many skin cells?
    a. 300 million
    b. 100 million
    c. 450 million
    d. 230 million

3. The skin is composed of how many primary layers?
    a. 6
    b. 3
    c. 4
    d. 9

4. What is Rosacea?
    a. A skin condition that causes blushing or visible blood vessels on the face
    b. When the immune system attacks the cells in the epidermis and the mucous membranes
    c. Patchy hair loss
    d. A condition that causes the skin to be dry, flaky, and bumpy

Dermatology Fun Facts

1. Humans shed around 40,000 skin cells every hour

2. Humans have hair follicles almost everywhere except for the palms of the hands, soles of the feet, and lips

3. The skin is a protective barrier from pathogens, chemicals, and UV rays. It helps regulate body temperature and prevents excessive water loss

4. Freckles are clusters of melanin, the pigment that gives color to the skin. They are most common in people with fair skin and they often darken with sun exposure

5. Fingernails grow three times faster than toenails

6. Human bodies have about 2-4 million sweat glands

Emergency Medicine

Emergency medicine is known as a medical specialty that deals with immense loads of pressure, speed, and thrill. It is a specialty focused on the care of patients who need immediate medical attention due to injuries or illnesses. Emergency medicine physicians are trained to handle a wide range of medical emergencies and provide effective care in high-pressure situations. They often work in the emergency departments of hospitals or in Urgent Care facilities. Their role is to evaluate and stabilize patients with life-threatening or urgent conditions. Emergency medicine physicians are trained to quickly assess patients, see if they need to be admitted into the hospital, diagnose their medical problems, and treat them appropriately. They treat a variety of patients who range from all ages and sizes. Emergency doctors immediately begin treatment when a patient has experienced trauma or is experiencing a serious medical issue. They handle more than one patient at a time and must prioritize them according to their symptoms. The patient who has life-endangering conditions takes first priority. They may see patients with stroke symptoms, chest pain, severe bleeding, head and spinal injuries, abdominal pain, and more. Being an emergency medicine physician comes with many key responsibilities. They must triage patients ensuring that those with life-threatening or critical injuries receive immediate attention first. They rapidly evaluate patients using physical examinations, diagnostic tests, and the patient's medical history. Next, they initiate treatment to stabilize their patients. This may include suturing (stitching) wounds, placing breathing tubes, or performing CPR. CPR stands for cardiopulmonary resuscitation. They work closely with other healthcare professionals like nurses, trauma surgeons, and other physicians to ensure coordinated care for the patient. Communication is a vital responsibility in any medical specialty. Emergency medicine physicians communicate with patients about their diagnosis and treatment plans. They speak with their patients' families to provide them with updates or give follow-up instructions. A crucial aspect of being an emergency physician is multi-tasking. They must be skilled at handling multiple patients at once while making rapid decisions. They adapt to changing situations in an unpredictable and fast-paced environment. It is important to note that emergency medicine doctors undergo special training during their residency to acquire the knowledge and skills necessary to manage a wide variety of urgent medical conditions. It can take up to 11 years of training and education to become an emergency medicine physician.

They begin with completing a bachelor's degree, usually in a science-related field. Common majors for students who want to go into medicine include neuroscience, biology, chemistry, psychology, and more. Then, in their third year of college or university, they must take the MCAT (Medical College Admissions Test) and apply for medical school. Applying for and gaining acceptance into medical school is a tough process. Excellent applications for medical school include volunteer hours, research projects, recommendation letters, clinical experience, and a high MCAT score. During the first two years of medical school, core subjects such as anatomy, biochemistry, and pharmacology are covered. During the last two years of medical school, there are clinical rotations in various medical specialties, which may include emergency medicine. Many medical specialties are covered during medical school, but if students wish to discover more, they may complete elective rotations. After completing medical school aspiring emergency medicine physicians need to apply for residency. Throughout medical school and the first years of residency, physicians must have completed all three parts of the USMLE (United States Medical Licensing Examination) or COMLEX (Comprehensive Osteopathic Medical Licensing Exam). There is currently about a 95% match rate for emergency medicine. Emergency medicine residency is 3-4 years in length. A strong application for residency includes high rotation grades, recommendation letters, and high exam grades. During residency, residents learn the aspects of emergency medicine, gain hands–on experience in diagnosing and treating patients, and work under experienced emergency medicine physicians. After completing residency, board certification is obtained by passing both a written and oral exam issued by the American Board of Emergency Medicine. The passing rate in 2022 was 95%. Just like board-certification, a fellowship is optional. They can pursue fellowship training in areas such as pediatric emergency medicine, critical care medicine, sports medicine, medical toxicology, and more. Becoming an emergency medicine physician requires at least 11 years of education and training after high school. Emergency medicine is a fast-paced and exciting specialty, which is very fulfilling. Emergency medicine physicians have the chance to save lives every day and are often the first doctors to treat patients during critical situations.

Why You Should Become an Emergency Medicine Physician

Diverse Patient Population

Emergency Medicine Physicians work with people of different ages, cultures, backgrounds, illnesses, and injuries

Fast-paced environment

If you enjoy working in a fast-paced environment or work well under pressure, emergency medicine might be right for you

First to see patients

In the Emergency Room, emergency medicine physicians are usually the first doctors to see and assess a patient

Decoding Medical Careers: A Teenage Guide to Medical Specialties

Emergency Medicine Trivia

1. Which of the following would most likely **not** see an emergency medicine doctor?
    a. A 65-year-old man showing heart attack symptoms
    b. A 40-year-old woman with injuries to her head and neck
    c. An 8-year-old boy with a cold and moderate ear pain
    d. A 15-year-old girl with severe abdominal pain

2. Which procedure would an emergency medicine doctor **most likely** perform?
    a. Appendectomy (removal of appendix)
    b. Tonsillectomy (removal of tonsils)
    c. Hysterectomy (removal of woman's uterus)
    d. Hip replacement

3. What is the medical term for the condition commonly known as a nosebleed?
    a. Rhinorrhea
    b. Nasal artery eruption
    c. Epistaxis
    d. Biopsy

4. You may have seen an AED before. What does it stand for?
    a. Automatic Erythema Detection
    b. Automated External Defibrillator
    c. Assisted Epilepsy Detection
    d. Aided Endocrine Defibrillator

All answers on next page

Emergency Medicine Trivia

1. Which of the following would most likely **not** see an emergency medicine doctor?
    a. A 65-year-old man showing heart attack symptoms
    b. A 40-year-old woman with injuries to her head and neck
    c. An 8-year-old boy with a cold and moderate ear pain
    d. A 15-year-old girl with severe abdominal pain

2. Which procedure would an emergency medicine doctor **most likely** perform?
    a. Appendectomy (removal of appendix)
    b. Tonsillectomy (removal of tonsils)
    c. Hysterectomy (removal of woman's uterus)
    d. Hip replacement

3. What is the medical term for the condition commonly known as a nosebleed?
    a. Rhinorrhea
    b. Nasal artery eruption
    c. Epistaxis
    d. Biopsy

4. You may have seen an AED before. What does it stand for?
    a. Automatic Erythema Detection
    b. Automated External Defibrillator
    c. Assisted Epilepsy Detection
    d. Aided Endocrine Defibrillator

Emergency Medicine Fun Facts

1. The busiest day for emergency rooms is Thanksgiving

2. In emergency rooms "Code Blue" is called when a patient requires resuscitation often due to respiratory or cardiac arrest

3. Emergency medicine doctors have encountered unusual objects removed from patients, light bulbs, toothbrushes, and sometimes live animals

4. The "trauma bay" in emergency rooms is where critically injured patients are treated

5. Appendicitis is the most common cause of acute abdominal pain for which you need surgery

Family Medicine

Family medicine is a specialty that focuses on treating and providing healthcare for patients of all ages, from newborns to the elderly. Family medicine doctors are also known as family physicians or general practitioners. They offer a wide range of medical services to patients in the context of family and community. They diagnose and treat common medical conditions, provide preventative care, and perform routine check-ups. Family medicine doctors can treat chronic conditions and evaluate a patient's symptoms to determine the next course of action. Additionally, they offer counseling on lifestyle modifications such as nutrition and mental health. The scope of family medicine is very broad. Family medicine physicians may perform minor surgical procedures, and offer prenatal (during and relating to pregnancy) and newborn care. They are trained to perform colonoscopies (procedure used to look inside the colon and rectum), endoscopies (procedure to look inside the body without performing major surgery), vasectomies (procedure to cut or tie tubes that carry sperm), suture lacerations, and more. All family medicine physicians are trained in obstetrics, meaning they can provide pre- and post-natal care, and deliver babies. They will coordinate with specialists when necessary, they may refer you to a cardiologist if they discover you have a heart murmur, or refer you to an ophthalmologist to treat issues with your eyesight. This ensures that the patient receives appropriate care. Family medicine is often confused with internal medicine. An internal medicine physician cares and treats adults, while family medicine physicians care for children, and adults, and often treat women's health issues. There are several subspecialties in family medicine which require additional training. Some of the following are adolescent medicine, pain medicine, sports medicine, and more. Family medicine physicians who specialize in adolescent medicine are trained in the diverse physical and mental characteristics of adolescents and manage their healthcare problems or issues. Family medicine physicians specialized in pain medicine treat patients experiencing severe pain due to an injury or illness. A core principle of family medicine is the continuity of care. The goal of family medicine physicians is to establish long-term relationships with their patients, they strive to understand their medical history and family dynamics. It's often said that family medicine physicians "grow with the family." They aim to provide personalized medical care to patients and their families throughout their lives.

The first step towards becoming a family medicine physician begins with obtaining a bachelor's degree and completing the prerequisites for medical school. The prerequisite courses for medical school include physics, biology, chemistry, organic chemistry, and biochemistry. Next, prepare for and take the MCAT (Medical College Admissions Test). The MCAT plays a large factor in gaining acceptance into medical school. The MCAT ranges from the lowest possible score being a 472 and the highest possible being a 528. An excellent application for medical school includes a high MCAT score, a strong GPA (Grade Point Average), volunteer hours, clinical experience, and recommendation letters from professors and peers. Once accepted into medical school, it typically takes four years to complete. Crucial skills are learnt during medical school, like how to examine and diagnose a patient. It is during the third and fourth years of medical school that students receive hands-on experience and learn clinical skills. Clinical rotations in medical school include internal medicine, OB/GYN, neurology, family medicine, surgery, and more. It is common to apply for residency early in the fourth year of medical school. Family medicine residency is known to be averagely competitive. The next step is to complete the intern year and residency. Family medicine residency lasts three years. During this period residents work with experienced family medicine physicians and are trained to diagnose and treat patients of all ages. Residency training is extremely in depth, it prepares a physician to begin their own career in their specialty. Throughout medical school and residency, physicians must take all three parts of the USMLE (United States Medical Licensing Exam) or COMLEX (Comprehensive Osteopathic Medical Licensing Exam). Many students and residents report that both exams are extremely challenging. After the completion of their residency, family medicine physicians can become board-certified by passing an exam by the American Board of Family Medicine. This exam tests doctors on everything they learned during medical school and residency. Family medicine physicians have the option to complete a fellowship after their residency, family medicine fellowships last 1-3 years. Some family medicine fellowships are sports medicine, pain medicine, and adolescent medicine which were discussed above. In order to begin practicing medicine in their location, family medicine physicians must obtain a license. Family medicine is an extremely patient-centered and diverse specialty that aims to care for patients of all ages and sizes.

Why You Should Become a Family Medicine Physician

High Income

Family medicine physicians make an average of $280,349+ a year

Patient Relationships

Family medicine physicians establish long-lasting and deep relationships with their patients

Job Satisfaction

75% of family medicine physicians report they are satisfied with their specialty and career

Patient Variety

Family medicine physicians treat people of all ages, sizes, and genders

Family Medicine Trivia

1. Family medicine physicians provide primary care and do not perform surgical procedures
    a. True
    b. False

2. What is the duration of a typical family medicine residency?
    a. 5 years
    b. 6 years
    c. 3 years
    d. 4 years

3. What is the medical term for the voicebox?
    a. The tibia
    b. The larynx
    c. The clavicle
    d. The hypothalamus

4. What is the hormone responsible for regulating sleep-wake cycles?
    a. Melatonin
    b. Insulin
    c. Progesterone
    d. Cortisol

All answers on next page

Family Medicine Trivia

1. Family medicine physicians provide primary care and do not perform surgical procedures
    a. True
    b. False

2. What is the duration of a typical family medicine residency?
    a. 5 years
    b. 6 years
    c. 3 years
    d. 4 years

3. What is the medical term for the voicebox?
    a. The tibia
    b. The larynx
    c. The clavicle
    d. The hypothalamus

4. What is the hormone responsible for regulating sleep-wake cycles?
    a. Melatonin
    b. Insulin
    c. Progesterone
    d. Cortisol

Family Medicine Fun Facts

1. Family Medicine physicians and primary care doctors can provide care for about 90% of a patient's healthcare needs

2. Family medicine doctors can work in a variety of settings including private practices, hospitals, and clinics

3. The competitiveness level for family medicine is relatively low

4. The average length of a family medicine appointment in the U.S. is 17 minutes

5. There is a growing need for osteopathic family medicine physicians

Gastroenterology

Gastroenterology is the medical specialty that focuses on the diagnosis and treatment of the digestive system. The digestive system includes organs such as the esophagus, stomach, small intestine, large intestine, liver, gallbladder, pancreas, and more. A gastroenterologist is an expert who specializes in conditions affecting the digestive system. "Gastro" means stomach, "entero" means intestines, and "ologist" means specialist. Gastroenterologists are skilled in the management of a wide range of gastrointestinal conditions, acute and chronic. They are able to distinguish normal gastrointestinal behavior from abnormal behavior. They understand the functions of the digestive system and its organs. Gastroenterologists may physically examine patients, insert a finger into their patient's rectum (stores waste from the colon), order blood and imaging tests, and perform endoscopic procedures. Overall, there are many key responsibilities a gastroenterologist has. They are trained to diagnose several digestive disorders and diseases, like lactose intolerance and heartburn. They use physical examinations, their patients' medical history, and tests to determine the cause of their symptoms. A patient may see a gastroenterologist if they are experiencing diverticulitis, abdominal pain, ulcers, vomiting, pancreatitis, and more. Gastroenterologists often perform endoscopic procedures. These procedures involve the use of a camera attached to a flexible tube to examine the inside of your body and detect any abnormalities. While using the endoscope, gastroenterologists can even obtain tissue samples for further analysis. Colonoscopies are known as the gold standard for colon cancer screening. Gastroenterologists have the opportunity to perform state-of-the-art procedures (like endoscopies and colonoscopies) without performing major surgery. After diagnosing a patient, gastroenterologists develop treatment plans for their patients. Treatment options may include dietary changes, medications, and in some cases surgery. Gastroenterologists work closely with other specialists such as surgeons and oncologists. Gastroenterologists manage conditions such as IBS (inflammatory bowel disease), Crohn's disease (inflammation in the digestive tract), ulcerative colitis (inflammation and ulcers on the lining of large intestine), celiac disease (immune reaction to eating gluten) and more. They monitor disease progression, adjust treatment plans, and strive to provide long-term care for their patients. Gastroenterology is also a research-oriented and evolving field. It is a field with advancements in technology and new treatments that are constantly being made.

Becoming a gastroenterologist begins with obtaining a bachelor's degree in a science-related field. Common majors for pre-medical students include biology, neuroscience, chemistry, physics, psychology, and more. College students typically take the MCAT (Medical College Acceptance Test) in their third year of school. The scoring on the MCAT ranges from 472 to 528. The MCAT is required to apply for medical school. After being accepted into medical school, it takes 4 years to complete. During medical school, you will earn a Doctor of Medicine (M.D) or Doctor of Osteopathic Medicine (D.O) degree. The first two years of medical school consist of lectures, lab work, and classroom-study. Core subjects such as anatomy, physiology, pharmacology, and medical ethics are covered. The last two years of medical school consist of clinical rotations in many medical specialties. These commonly include internal medicine, neurology, surgery, OB/GYN, cardiology, and ophthalmology. If students want to gain hands-on experience in other specialties, they can complete elective rotations. Students apply and match into residency in their fourth year of medical school. Aspiring gastroenterologists must complete a 3-year residency in internal medicine. During the residency, they will gain practical experience, treat patients, perform procedures, and work with experienced physicians. An internal medicine residency in the foundation for further specialization in the digestive tract. Throughout medical school and residency, physicians must complete all three parts of the USMLE (United States Medical Licensing Exam) or COMLEX (Comprehensive Osteopathic Medical Licensing Exam). After completing residency, gastroenterologists pursue a fellowship in gastroenterology, which lasts another three years. During their fellowship gastroenterologists practice endoscopic procedures, participate in patient care, and become experts in the field of gastroenterology. They also thoroughly examine, diagnose, and treat all the different kinds of digestive diseases. Gastroenterology is one of the most competitive internal medicine fellowships. Following the completion of their fellowship, gastroenterologists become board-certified by taking an exam by the ABIM (American Board of Internal Medicine) or by the AOBIM (American Osteopathic Board of Internal Medicine). Board-certification is not required, but it showcases a physician's expertise in their field. Subspecializing in gastroenterology is optional, but gastroenterologists may choose to specialize in hepatology (treatment of liver diseases and conditions), advanced endoscopy, irritable bowel disease, gastrointestinal oncology, and more. Overall, gastroenterology is a broad field that covers the entire digestive system, and also the pancreas and liver! The field of gastroenterology demands years of schooling, training, and experience.

Why You Should Become a Gastroenterologist

Don't like the idea of surgery?
Gastroenterologists commonly perform procedures, not surgery

High Salary
Gastroenterologists make an average of $411,070 a year

In Demand
Gastroenterology was ranked the most "in-demand" specialty in 2021

Teamwork
Gastroenterologists interact with other physicians, patients, and colleagues very often

Gastroenterology Trivia

1. What is the largest internal organ in the human body?
    a. Large intestine
    b. Skin
    c. Liver
    d. Kidney

2. The small intestine is longer than the large intestine.
    a. True
    b. False

3. The ____ produces insulin, the hormone that regulates blood sugar levels
    a. Kidney
    b. Pancreas
    c. Liver
    d. Small intestine

4. Which organ stores bile, a fluid that is made by the liver?
    a. Bladder
    b. Gallbladder
    c. Esophagus
    d. Kidney

All answers on next page

Gastroenterology Trivia

1. What is the largest internal organ in the human body?
    a. Large intestine
    b. Skin
    c. Liver
    d. Kidney

2. The small intestine is longer than the large intestine.
    a. True
    b. False

3. The ____ produces insulin, the hormone that regulates blood sugar levels
    a. Kidney
    b. Pancreas
    c. Liver
    d. Small intestine

4. Which organ stores bile, a fluid made by the liver?
    a. Bladder
    b. Gallbladder
    c. Esophagus
    d. Kidney

Gastroenterology Fun Facts

1. The small intestine is 22 feet in length

2. It generally takes 24 to 72 hours to move through the digestive tract

3. The human digestive system produces 0.5-1.5 liters of saliva every day to help with digestion

4. The liver has a unique ability to regenerate itself, a liver can regenerate to normal size even if 90% is removed

5. Platypuses don't have stomachs

6. The average adult stomach can hold 4-8 pounds of food

General Surgery

General surgery is the medical specialty that focuses on the surgical treatment of a wide range of conditions affecting different organs and systems in the body. The Cambridge English Dictionary defines surgery as "the treatment of injuries and diseases by cutting the body open to repair or remove the damaged parts." General surgeons are highly skilled and trained professionals who perform a variety of surgical procedures to treat their patient's health issues. Appendectomies, cholecystectomies (removal of gallbladder), hernia repairs, and more, are all done by general surgeons. General surgeons have extensive knowledge of the digestive tract, the endocrine system, the blood vessels and heart, surgical oncology, the abdomen, and more. There are several key aspects of what general surgeons do. They are trained to handle a broad scope of surgical procedures, rather than focusing on a specific area of the body. They will often be involved in surgeries on the abdomen, gastrointestinal tract, endocrine system, liver, and more. General surgeons assess patients, order appropriate tests, interpret the results, and determine the right surgical course of action. General surgeons are responsible for the preoperative, operative, and postoperative care of their patients. Some tests a general surgeon may order are chest X-rays, electrocardiograms, CT scans (imaging test), MRIs, and blood tests. They also play a vital role in emergency surgeries and trauma cases. A general surgeon may operate on an appendix about to rupture and emergency hernia surgeries. They perform life-saving procedures on patients with serious conditions. General surgeons often work closely with other medical professionals. They may collaborate with urologists, gastroenterologists, and oncologists to provide the best care for their patients. They also work with surgical techs, anesthesiologists , and scrub nurses inside the operating room. General surgeons are often known as "surgical know-it-alls" because of their knowledge in all aspects of surgery. They have the ability to showcase their broad knowledge and experience in the operating room, where they will spend much of their time. The operating room can be described as a large, sterile environment, equipped with all the necessary tools for surgery. It is filled with high-tech equipment and monitors which are used by the several doctors and staff who are inside the operating room. Before general surgeons begin surgery, they must "scrub in." This means washing their hands and forehands to become sterile before beginning surgery. General surgeons truly are "know-it-alls" inside the operating room, they save lives everyday, and play an immense role to all of their patients by improving their quality of life.

Becoming a general surgeon begins just as any other medical specialty with obtaining a bachelor's degree. It is important to maintain a high GPA (Grade Point Average) and to take the prerequisite courses for medical school. The prerequisite courses for medical school include physics, biology, chemistry, organic chemistry, and biochemistry classes. Students typically take the MCAT (Medical College Admissions Test) in their third year of college or university. A high MCAT score is crucial for gaining acceptance into medical school. Once accepted into medical school, it will take four years to complete. The first two years of medical school focus on subjects such as anatomy, physiology, pharmacology, and medical ethics. The last two years of medical school focus on clinical rotations, where students gain hands-on experience in different medical specialties, like surgery. Throughout medical school, students will have to take several challenging exams. Following medical school, aspiring general surgeons must complete a general surgery residency. General surgery residency takes five years to complete, yet some programs require an extra two mandatory research years. General surgery interns don't spend much time in the operating room, junior residents have the opportunity to perform minor operations, and senior residents perform complex operations with less supervision. During general surgery residency, residents practice scrubbing in, suturing, and performing surgical procedures. After the completion of residency, general surgeons can become board certified by passing an exam by the American Board of Surgery. It is a 300-question exam that lasts 8 hours, it tests a surgeon's knowledge of general surgical principles. Board-certification is not mandatory, but many physicians choose or want to become board-certified. General surgeons may choose to specialize further and complete a fellowship. Some general surgery fellowships are pediatric surgery, surgical oncology, hand surgery, colorectal surgery, and more. Finally, in order to begin practicing medicine in their location, general surgeons must obtain a license. Like all medical professionals, general surgeons must continue learning and staying updated on the latest advancements in their specialty to provide the best care for their patients. General surgery is an extremely broad specialty that works with all kinds of injuries and ailments. It is a perfect specialty for someone who craves diversity and loves the operating room.

Why You Should Become a General Surgeon

High Salary

General surgeons were ranked #4 of the highest paying jobs in 2023

Valuable Skills

As a general surgeon, you learn the skills of communication, problem-solving, teamwork, and hand-eye coordination

Respected Profession

General surgeons are highly respected and are experts in the operating room

Challenges

General surgeons deal with puzzling patient cases and perform complex procedures

General Surgery Trivia

1. What type of surgery involves the removal of the spleen?
    a. Splenectomy
    b. Abdominectomy
    c. Whipple surgery
    d. Cholecystectomy

2. Which medical specialty is focused on the treatment of diseases and conditions of the brain and nervous system?
    a. Orthopedic surgery
    b. Neurosurgery
    c. Plastic surgery
    d. Internal medicine

3. What is the surgical procedure to remove part or all of the thyroid gland?
    a. Appendectomy
    b. Hysterectomy
    c. Thyroidectomy
    d. Colectomy

4. What is the surgical specialty that deals with disorders of the bones, joints, and muscles?
    a. Ophthalmology
    b. Trauma surgery
    c. Urology
    d. Orthopedic surgery

All answers on next page

General Surgery Trivia

1. What type of surgery involves the removal of the spleen?
    a. Splenectomy
    b. Abdominectomy
    c. Whipple surgery
    d. Cholecystectomy

2. Which medical specialty is focused on the treatment of diseases and conditions on the brain and nervous system?
    a. Orthopedic Surgery
    b. Neurosurgery
    c. Plastic surgery
    d. Internal medicine

3. What is the surgical procedure to remove part or all of the thyroid gland?
    a. Appendectomy
    b. Hysterectomy
    c. Thyroidectomy
    d. Colectomy

4. What is the surgical specialty that deals with disorders of the bones, joints, and muscles?
    a. Ophthalmology
    b. Trauma surgery
    c. Urology
    d. Orthopedic surgery

General Surgery Fun Facts

1. Dr. Joseph Lister developed antiseptics, which prevented infections in wounds during and after surgery. He is considered a pioneer of infection control

2. Surgical robots have become increasingly popular in modern surgery, they allow for more precision and visualization during surgery

3. The kidney was the first human organ to be transplanted successfully in 1954

4. Dr. Henry Heimlich was an American thoracic surgeon who invented the Heimlich maneuver

5. Surgeons often wear green and blue scrubs in the operating room to reduce eye strain

Internal Medicine

Internal medicine is a medical specialty that focuses on the prevention, diagnosis, and treatment of various diseases and medical conditions in adults. Internal medicine physicians are commonly known as internists. They are specially trained to solve diagnostic problems and manage severe illnesses or diseases. There is a special complexity and uniqueness to internal medicine. The American College of Physicians says that "internal medicine physicians see the big picture." Internal medicine physicians undergo extensive training to become experts in diagnosing and treating diseases affecting internal organs and systems. They understand how everything in the human body works in unison. The thing that distinguishes internal medicine from family medicine and pediatrics is that they focus on adult care. Internists are also known as "diagnostic detectives" as they are able to diagnose and treat patients who may present with multiple and unclear symptoms. Internal medicine doctors can treat a broad range of health issues. Patients experiencing hypertension (high blood pressure), asthma, osteoporosis, ear infections, bronchitis, and more, can see an internal medicine physician to be treated. According to the American Medical Association, "internists have a great understanding of disease prevention, mental health, substance abuse, and common problems of the nervous system and reproductive organs." They are also trained to serve in multiple settings. Internists can provide inpatient and outpatient care, meaning that they can work in hospitals and clinics. At a routine internal medicine appointment, the physician may check their patient's vital signs, review their medical history, examine their ears, mouth, and eyes, check their posture, and more. If necessary, internal medicine physicians may refer their patients to another specialist for further evaluation. For example, if a patient informs their doctor about a suspicious mole they found on their body, their doctor may refer them to a dermatologist. For adults, an internal medicine physician is usually the first doctor they see or express any health issues to, which is why it is necessary to refer them to appropriate specialists. There are many subspecialties of internal medicine which include gastroenterology, nephrology, oncology, endocrinology, hematology, and more. A goal of internists is to build deep relationships with their patients and to provide them with care throughout their adulthoods. Overall, internal medicine is a highly unique specialty with expert doctors who play an immense role in healthcare.

Becoming an internal medicine physician begins just as any other medical specialty with obtaining a bachelor's degree. During undergraduate studies, it is important to maintain a strong academic record. Students typically take the MCAT (Medical College Acceptance Test) in their third year of college or university. A high MCAT score is crucial for gaining acceptance into medical school, which is a rigorous process. Once accepted into medical school, it takes four years to complete. In the first two years of medical school, students learn key subjects such as anatomy, physiology, biochemistry, and pathology. In the last two years of medical school, students complete clinical rotations in various medical specialties, including internal medicine. Students receive hands-on experience, learn how to take medical histories and work under the supervision of experienced physicians. It is in the third or fourth year of medical school that students apply for residency. A residency application requires a USMLE (United States Medical Licensing Examination) or COMLEX (Comprehensive Osteopathic Medical Licensing Examination) score. Once matched into internal medicine residency, it takes three years to complete. Internal medicine is ranked as one of the least competitive residencies. During residency, residents become well-versed in all areas of internal medicine. Internal medicine residency is very diverse, it covers areas of cardiology, gastroenterology, dermatology, ophthalmology, and more. Residency is very in-depth, it trains a physician to have knowledge in all areas of their specialty. After completing an internal medicine residency, physicians can become board-certified by passing an exam issued by the ABIM (American Board of Internal Medicine) or the AOBIM (American Osteopathic Board of Internal Medicine). The difference between MDs and DOs is that MDs take a more medication-focused approach to medicine, while DOs take a more holistic approach to medicine. Internal medicine physicians often consider pursuing a subspecialty such as gastroenterology, endocrinology, cardiology, infectious disease, and more. These fellowships are optional, but typically take 2-3 years to complete. The complete process of becoming an internal medicine physician takes 11 years. This process requires a significant commitment to education and training.

Why You Should Become an Internal Medicine Physician

Subspecialties

There are a number of subspecialties following internal medicine such as gastroenterology, cardiology, endocrinology, and more

In Demand

Internal medicine is among the most in-demand physician specialties

High Salary

The average internal medicine doctor in the U.S. makes $238,100+ a year

Detective Work

They are trained to diagnose and treat multiple and unclear symptoms, which is highly fulfilling

Decoding Medical Careers: A Teenage Guide to Medical Specialties

Internal Medicine Trivia

1. What is the normal range for blood pressure in adults?
    a. 90/60
    b. 120/80
    c. 180/110
    d. 180/120

2. What is the medical term for inflammation of the liver?
    a. Hepatitis
    b. Inflammatory liver syndrome
    c. Gastritis
    d. Fatty liver disease

3. What is the medical term for an abnormal heartbeat or irregular heart rhythm?
    a. Angina
    b. Cardiomyopathy
    c. Arrhythmia
    d. Cardiac arrest

4. What is the medical term known as a sideways curvature of the spine?
    a. Osteoporosis
    b. Osteomyelitis
    c. Scoliosis
    d. Arthritis

All answers on next page

Internal Medicine Trivia

1. What is the normal range for blood pressure in adults?
    a. 90/60
    b. 120/80
    c. 180/110
    d. 180/120

2. What is the medical term for inflammation of the liver?
    a. Hepatitis
    b. Inflammatory liver syndrome
    c. Gastritis
    d. Fatty liver disease

3. What is the medical term for an abnormal heartbeat or irregular heart rhythm?
    a. Angina
    b. Cardiomyopathy
    c. Arrhythmia
    d. Cardiac arrest

4. What is the medical term known as a sideways curvature of the spine?
    a. Osteoporosis
    b. Osteomyelitis
    c. Scoliosis
    d. Arthritis

Internal Medicine Fun Facts

1. Sir William Osler is a prominent figure in the history of medicine, he is often known as "the father of internal medicine"

2. National Internal Medicine Day is on October 28th

3. The American Board of Internal Medicine was established in 1936

4. Doctors who specialize in both internal medicine and pediatrics are called "Med-Peds"

5. Internists are often known as the "doctor's doctor" because other physicians often seek their professional advice and guidance

Nephrology

Nephrology is the medical specialty that focuses on the diagnosis and treatment of diseases related to the kidneys. The kidneys are two bean-shaped organs that filter blood, remove waste, extra water, and electrolytes to make urine. The kidneys play a crucial role in maintaining the human body's overall health by filtering waste, regulating blood pressure, keeping the bones healthy, and balancing electrolytes. Nephrologists are medical doctors who have specialized training in this field and are experts in understanding the structure, function, and disorders of the kidney and its associated systems. They recognize how the kidney's conditions affect the rest of the body. Nephrologists are responsible for diagnosing and managing various kidney-related conditions. They can treat patients with all stages of kidney disease, they can help treat kidney stones, manage hypertension, kidney transplants, and more. A crucial role of nephrologists is to supervise dialysis. Dialysis is a type of treatment to help the kidneys remove extra fluid and waste products from the blood when they can no longer function on their own. When the kidneys cannot function on their own, a kidney transplant may be considered. Nephrologists also participate in the kidney transplant process, they care for the patient receiving and giving the kidney. Transplant nephrology requires an extra year of training through a transplant nephrology fellowship. Common conditions and diseases that a nephrologist may treat are high blood pressure, kidney stones, nephrotic syndrome (kidneys release too much protein in urine), UTIs (urinary tract infections), kidney infections, and more. In order to diagnose and treat these conditions a nephrologist may order several tests and imaging scans. These include CT scans, X-rays, kidney function tests, blood tests, and urine tests. The differences between nephrologists and urologists are commonly unclear. Nephrologists specialize in conditions and diseases that affect the kidneys. Urologists specialize in issues related to the urinary and reproductive systems. This includes the bladder, penis, testicles, urethra, and urinary tract. Another key difference is that nephrologists do not perform surgery, instead, they perform procedures. Procedures that a nephrologist can perform are dialysis, kidney biopsies, and more. Urologists have surgical training and can perform a number of surgeries. The best physician to see regarding concerns about your kidneys or kidney function is a nephrologist. They are experts in all issues related to the kidneys. Nephrologists have the adequate training, education, and experience to treat even the most complex kidney conditions.

Becoming a nephrologist begins with completing a bachelor's degree in a science-related field. It is important to be aware of the GPA (Grade Point Average) requirements for medical school and to be involved in extracurricular activities or research projects. Students will need an MCAT (Medical College Admissions Test) score to apply to medical school. The lowest possible score on the MCAT is 472, and the highest possible is 528. After being accepted into medical school it will take 4 years to complete. The four years of medical school combine classroom study and clinical rotations in various medical specialties. The first two years include classroom study and the last two years include clinical rotations in several medical specialties. Students typically rotate through internal medicine, surgery, neurology, psychiatry and more. If students wish to discover or experience specialties that their program did not cover, they can complete elective rotations. Students usually apply for residency in their third or fourth year of medical school. Aspiring nephrologists must pass all three stages of the USMLE (United States Medical Licensing Examination) or COMLEX (Comprehensive Osteopathic Medical Licensing Exam). Nephrologists complete a three-year residency in internal medicine. Internal medicine residency prepares nephrologists for further specialization in kidney care during fellowship. It provides residents with practical experience in diagnosing and treating a wide range of medical conditions. Nephrologists need to complete a 2-3 year fellowship after their residency. During the fellowship, physicians receive specialized training in nephrology, focusing on kidney disorders, transplantation, dialysis, and related areas. The kidney is an intricate structure, during fellowships nephrologists focus their medical skills toward the kidneys. After they have completed their training, nephrologists have the option to become board-certified. Board certification is not required, but having a license is. Board certification can be achieved by passing an exam by the ABIM (American Board of Internal Medicine) or through the AOBIM (American Osteopathic Board of Internal Medicine). In order to begin practicing medicine in their location, physicians must obtain a license. Nephrologists must then stay updated on the latest findings and treatments within their field. It is important to be aware of the advancements in their specialty so they can offer the best treatments available to their patients. Overall, nephrology is a complex specialty with a minimum of 13 years of training following the completion of high school.

Why You Should Become a Nephrologist

Life-saving procedures

Nephrologists perform life-saving procedures like dialysis and supervise kidney transplants

High Salary

The average salary of a nephrologist is $308,0208 annually

Continuity of Care

Nephrologists have patients whom they will see for long periods of time

Intellectually stimulating

Nephrologists have a challenging work environment, many physicians argue that nephrologists are some of the smartest doctors

Decoding Medical Careers: A Teenage Guide to Medical Specialties

Nephrology Trivia

1. True or false: You only need one kidney to survive
    a. True
    b. False

2. What is the common name for the hard mineral deposits that can form in the kidneys?
    a. Kidney minerality
    b. Kidney stones
    c. Kidney cysts
    d. Nephroticitis

3. Which of the following is a symptom of kidney stones?
    a. Toothache
    b. Dizziness
    c. Runny nose
    d. Back pain

4. What is the tiny filtering unit of the kidney called?
    a. Neuron
    b. Cells
    c. Nephron
    d. Hemoglobin

All answers on next page

Nephrology Trivia

1. True or false: You only need one kidney to survive
    a. True
    b. False

2. What is the common name for the hard mineral deposits that can form in the kidneys?
    a. Kidney minerality
    b. Kidney stones
    c. Kidney cysts
    d. Nephroticitis

3. Which of the following is a symptom of kidney stones?
    a. Toothache
    b. Dizziness
    c. Runny nose
    d. Back pain

4. What is the tiny filtering unit of the kidney called?
    a. Neuron
    b. Cells
    c. Nephron
    d. Hemoglobin

Nephrology Fun Facts

1. World Kidney Day is on March 14th

2. The first successful kidney transplant was performed in 1954 by Dr. Joseph Murray

3. The world's largest kidney stone was about the size of a grapefruit and as long as a banana

4. Each kidney contains around 1 million filtering units called nephrons

5. In ancient times, people associated the kidneys with their conscience and feelings

6. Horseshoe kidney is when the kidneys are fused together, it occurs in about 1 in 500 children

Neurology & Neurosurgery

Neurology is the branch of medicine that focuses on the study and treatment of disorders of the nervous system. There are two main parts of the nervous system. The central nervous system is made up of the brain and spinal cord. The peripheral nervous system is made up of nerves that branch out from the spinal cord and extend throughout the body. The nervous system is severely complex and impacts every aspect of a human's well-being. A neurologist is a medical doctor who specializes in this field. A neurologist has extensive knowledge of the anatomy, function, and conditions of the nervous system. They are trained to diagnose and treat a wide range of neurological conditions, both acute and chronic. Neurologists use their knowledge and expertise to recognize conditions such as epilepsy, Parkinson's disease, Alzheimer's disease, cerebral palsy, and more. In order to diagnose and treat their patients neurologists must conduct thorough neurological exams. These include asking about their patient's medical history, examining their coordination, muscle strength, motor function and balance, reflexes, sensation, and more. Neurologists may also conduct several tests to determine what is wrong with their patient. An electroencephalogram measures brain activity. A cerebrospinal fluid analysis involves taking a sample of fluid from the brain and spine. An angiogram shows if blood vessels are blocked or abnormal. The results of neurological tests influence the treatment plan. After making a diagnosis neurologists develop treatment plans like prescribing medications, physical therapy, lifestyle modifications, or surgery. It is important to note that neurologists do not perform surgery, neurosurgeons perform surgery. Neurosurgery is the medical specialty that focuses on the surgical treatment of disorders and conditions affecting the nervous system. Neurosurgeons are medical professionals who undergo extensive training to perform complex surgical procedures on the brain and nervous system. Although they are surgeons, they can provide both surgical and non-surgical treatment to their patients. Neurologists and neurosurgeons work closely together, a neurologist may refer their patients to a neurosurgeon for further evaluation or treatment. A neurosurgeon can perform various complex surgeries and procedures which include craniotomies (removal of part of the skull bone for access into the brain), laminectomies (removal of part or all of the vertebral bone), tumor removal, spinal fusion (surgery to connect two or more bones in the spine), and many more. Neurosurgeons and neurologists have much in common, and are both experts in the diagnosis and treatment of the brain and nervous system.

On the path to becoming a neurologist, one must undertake a challenging, rewarding, and specialized journey of education. It begins with attending a 4-year college or university and graduating with a degree in a science-related field. It is important to take the required classes for medical school. Maintaining a high GPA and being involved in extracurriculars will increase a student's chances of being accepted into medical school. Students typically take the MCAT (Medical College Admissions Test) in their third year of college or university. The MCAT tests students on their problem-solving skills, critical thinking, and the basic sciences. Once accepted into medical school it will take four years to earn an M.D (Medical Doctor) or D.O (Doctor of Osteopathic Medicine) degree. The first two years of medical school focus on classroom study and subjects such as anatomy, pharmacology, and the basics of patient care. After their second year of medical school, students take the USMLE (United States Medical Licensing Examination) or COMLEX (Comprehensive Osteopathic Medical Licensing Exam). The last two years of medical school are centered on clinical rotations in many medical specialties (including neurology) and learning how to perform patient procedures. Following medical school, aspiring neurologists complete their first year of residency in internal medicine. The first year of residency is called the intern year. The last three years of residency are focused on neurology. Neurology residents receive specialized training in diagnosing and treating neurological conditions. Neurologists may consider pursuing a fellowship after completing residency. Some neurology fellowship subspecialties include pediatric neurology, vascular neurology, brain injury medicine, epilepsy, and more. These fellowships are commonly 1-2 years in length. Neurologists can become board certified through the American Board of Psychiatry and Neurology. Although board certification is not mandatory, it can demonstrate a neurologist's expertise in their field. Neurosurgeons complete the same training as neurologists, but undergo a longer and much more specialized residency program. They obtain a bachelor's degree at college or university, and take the MCAT. After completing their pre-medical education, they apply for medical school. Neurosurgeons receive the same education as neurologists during medical school. After completing medical school, aspiring neurosurgeons must apply for residency. The first year of neurosurgery residency begins with a one-year internship in general surgery. Following their internship, residents complete a 5-7 year residency in a neurosurgery program. After residency, neurosurgeons can consider pursuing a fellowship and becoming board-certified.

Why You Should Become a Neurologist or Neurosurgeon

Respected Profession

Neurologists and neurosurgeons specialize in one of the most important systems in the body

High Salary

Neurologists make $307,100 a year and neurosurgeons can make up to $746,601 a year

Interesting Surgeries

Neurosurgeons have the opportunity to perform a wide range of challenging and unique surgeries

Exciting Work

Neurologists work with intricate diseases and conditions

Nervous System Trivia

1. Which part of the brain regulates heart rhythm, breathing, blood flow, and oxygen levels?

    a. Neurons

    b. The frontal lobe

    c. The Medulla

    d. The temporal lobe

2. Which part of the brain manages conscious thoughts, meaning, and things you do?

    a. The cerebrum

    b. The occipital lobe

    c. The brain stem

    d. The temporal lobe

3. Which brain disease is characterized by a growing loss of memory and cognitive function?

    a. Epilepsy

    b. Alzheimer's disease

    c. Parkinson's disease

    d. Meningitis

4. Which part of the brain manages taste, hearing, sight, touch, and smell?

    a. The parietal lobe

    b. The spinal cord

    c. The frontal lobe

    d. The occipital lobe

All answers on next page

Nervous System Trivia

1. Which part of the brain regulates heart rhythm, breathing, blood flow, and oxygen levels?
    a. Neurons
    b. The frontal lobe
    c. The Medulla
    d. The temporal lobe

2. Which part of the brain manages conscious thoughts, meaning, and things you do?
    a. The cerebrum
    b. The occipital lobe
    c. The brain stem
    d. The temporal lobe

3. Which brain disease is characterized by a growing loss of memory and cognitive function?
    a. Epilepsy
    b. Alzheimer's disease
    c. Parkinson's disease
    d. Meningitis

4. Which part of the brain manages taste, hearing, sight, touch, and smell?
    a. The parietal lobe
    b. The spinal cord
    c. The frontal lobe
    d. The occipital lobe

Neuro Fun Facts

1. The brain can not feel pain because it has no pain receptors

2. The average adult human brain weighs about 3 pounds

3. 60% of the human brain is made up of fat, making it the fattiest organ in the human body

4. The brain finishes developing and forming in a person's mid-late 20s

5. The human brain consists of about 86 billion neurons

6. During some brain operations, patients may be required to stay awake

Obstetrics & Gynecology

Obstetrics and Gynecology is the medical specialty that focuses on the care of the female reproductive system. The female reproductive system is made up of the uterus, fallopian tubes, vagina, vulva, and cervix. The female reproductive system allows a woman to produce eggs, and when one is fertilized the reproductive system will protect and nourish it until it is fully developed. Obstetrics involves the management of pregnancy, childbirth, and postpartum care. Gynecology is the study and treatment of diseases and disorders of the female reproductive system. Not every obstetrician is also a gynecologist, and vice versa. But, OB/GYNs are doctors who specialize in both obstetrics and gynecology. There are several key aspects to obstetrics and gynecology. OB/GYNs care for pregnant women and ensure they have a safe pregnancy. They monitor the mother and fetus throughout the pregnancy and provide prenatal evaluations. OB/GYNs can assist with vaginal deliveries and perform cesarean sections. They can manage high-risk pregnancies and complications during labor. They have quick-thinking skills which allow them to work under pressure in the event where complications arise. The gynecology aspect of obstetrics and gynecology includes treating issues related to the female reproductive organs. Patients experiencing menstrual irregularities, pelvic pain, endometriosis, PCOS (polycystic ovary syndrome), STIs (sexually transmitted infections), infertility and more can all see an OB/GYN to address their health issues. OB/GYNs counsel and assist women in family planning decisions. They can provide birth control options, which include pills, intrauterine devices (IUDs), implants, and shots. They can offer guidance on fertility options and treatments for women trying to conceive. OB/GYNs are surgeons and can perform a range of surgeries. Common operations an OB/GYN may conduct are hysterectomies (removal of the uterus), myomectomies (removal of uterine fibroids), ovarian cystectomies, uterine polypectomy (removal of uterine polyps), and more. OB/GYNs play a large role in preventative care. They perform regular screenings for cervical cancer (pap smear), and breast exams. They can administer vaccines such as the human papillomavirus (HPV) vaccine to protect against certain diseases. As women grow older and reach menopause OB/GYNs can help them control the symptoms associated with menopause. Some of the symptoms include hot flashes, trouble sleeping, moodiness, irritability, and depression. In summary, OB/GYNs play a vital role in promoting and maintaining the reproductive health of women at different stages of life.

Becoming an OB/GYN is a journey of education, training, and dedication to women's health at all stages of life. It begins with obtaining a bachelor's degree and fulfilling the prerequisite courses for medical school. The prerequisite courses for medical school include biology, physics, biochemistry, English, organic chemistry, and more. Students typically take the MCAT (Medical College Admissions Test) in their third year of college or university. The MCAT is a difficult exam that requires months to prepare for. A strong medical school application includes a high MCAT score, participation in volunteer work, healthcare experience, and a well-rounded academic record. Once accepted into medical school, it typically takes four years to complete. Completing medical school with an M.D. or D.O. degree is mandatory to become an OB/GYN. The difference between the two is that MDs take a more medication-focused approach to medicine while DOs take a more holistic approach to medicine. During the final years of medical school, students complete clinical rotations in several specialties, including obstetrics and gynecology. Before residency, medical students take the USMLE (United States Medical Licensing Examination) or COMLEX (Comprehensive Osteopathic Medical Licensing Examination) Steps 1 and 2. After graduating from medical school, physicians must undergo a residency to gain expertise in their field. In recent years, the competitiveness of obstetrics and gynecology has increased. An OB/GYN residency is 4 years in length. During residency OB/GYNs receive specialized training in all aspects of obstetrics and gynecology. This includes labor and delivery, surgery, prenatal care, family planning, disease prevention, and more. During residency, residents perform numerous deliveries, perform many hysterectomies, perform pelvic exams, and much more. During residency, residents take the USMLE or COMLEX Step 3 exam. After the completion of their residency, OB/GYNs can become board-certified by passing an exam issued by the American Board of Obstetrics and Gynecology. Also after the completion of their residency, OB/GYNs may choose to pursue a fellowship. Subspecialties in obstetrics and gynecology include gynecologic oncology, maternal-fetal medicine, reproductive endocrinology and infertility, and more. Lastly, OB/GYNs must obtain a license to begin practicing medicine in their location. Throughout their careers, OB/GYNs need to continue their education and stay up to date with the latest procedures and advancements. Obstetrics and gynecology is a challenging yet rewarding field that requires hard work, a passion for women's health, and determination.

Why You Should Become an OB/GYN

Variety of tasks

OB/GYNs can perform surgery, perform routine screenings, deliver babies, and help with reproductive issues

Subspecialties

There are several subspecialties for OB/GYNs allowing them to further specialize

Personal Fulfillment

OB/GYNs bring life into the world and help others with their health issues

Job Stability

There is a constant need for OB/GYNs

Decoding Medical Careers: A Teenage Guide to Medical Specialties

OB/GYN Trivia

1. Which of the following is a condition that causes pelvic pain due to the lining of the uterus growing outside of it?

    a. Menstruation

    b. Endometriosis

    c. Uterine fibroids

    d. PCOS

2. During labor and delivery, what is the term for the baby's position when the head is facing down and the baby is ready to be born?

    a. Breech

    b. Vertex

    c. Dilated

    d. Cephalic

3. Which famous TV show features a redheaded, double-board certified OB/GYN subspecializing in maternal-fetal surgery?

    a. Greys Anatomy

    b. The Big Bang Theory

    c. Chicago Med

    d. The Resident

4. On average, how much does a baby weigh after birth?

    a. 9-10 pounds

    b. 6-7 pounds

    c. 4-5 pounds

    d. 3-4 pounds

All answers on next page

OB/GYN Trivia

1. Which of the following is a condition that causes pelvic pain due to the lining of the uterus growing outside of it?
    a. Menstruation
    b. Endometriosis
    c. Uterine fibroids
    d. PCOS

2. During labor and delivery, what is the term for the baby's position when the head is facing down and the baby is ready to be born?
    a. Breech
    b. Vertex
    c. Dilated
    d. Cephalic

3. Which famous TV show features a redheaded, double-board certified OB/GYN subspecializing in maternal-fetal medicine?
    a. Greys Anatomy
    b. The Big Bang Theory
    c. Chicago Med
    d. The Resident

4. On average, how much does a baby weigh after birth?
    a. 9-10 pounds
    b. 6-7 pounds
    c. 4-5 pounds
    d. 3-4 pounds

OB/GYN Fun Facts

1. George Nicholas Papanicolaou invented the Pap smear, a test for detecting cervical cancer

2. Louise Joy Brown was the world's first baby to be conceived via IVF (in vitro fertilization)

3. After giving birth, many mothers experience the "birthing blues"

4. At birth, the normal female ovary has about 1-2 million eggs

5. Studies suggest that women living or spending lots of time together may experience synchronization of their menstrual cycles, it is called the "McClintock effect"

Oncology

Oncology is the branch of medicine that deals with the prevention, diagnosis, and treatment of cancer. Cancer is defined as a disease caused by an uncontrolled growth of cells in a part of the body. An oncologist is a doctor who specializes in diagnosing and treating cancer. Oncologists help and manage cancer patients throughout their challenging journey. They can diagnose cancer, design treatment plans, oversee cancer treatment, and manage a patient's symptoms. Oncologists are skilled in interpreting medical tests, imaging studies, blood tests, and can perform biopsies. Biopsies are procedures to remove a piece of tissue or a sample of cells so it can be tested in a laboratory. They can be used to diagnose the presence and type of cancer in a patient. Once a diagnosis is confirmed, an oncologist can determine the extent and spread of the cancer through a process called staging. Most cancers have four stages, the higher the number, the more cancer has spread throughout the body. Oncologists create personalized treatment plans for each of their patients based on factors such as the type of cancer, its stage, and the patient's overall health. Some of the main cancer treatments include chemotherapy, radiation therapy, immunotherapy, hormone therapy, and surgery. Oncologists will discuss treatment options with their patients and review each option's benefits and side effects. The main cancer treatment side effects are anemia, nausea, vomiting, and fatigue. As part of their job, oncologists will monitor their patients throughout their treatment and provide them with support. Regular check-ups and tests are necessary to ensure the effectiveness of the treatment and to detect any complications. There are several types of oncologists. Surgical oncologists can remove tumors and cancerous tissue, and they will help their patients recover from surgery. Medical oncologists treat cancer using chemotherapy, immunotherapy, and more. They are known as the "primary cancer doctors." Radiation oncologists use radiation therapy to treat their patient's cancer. Gynecologic oncologists treat cervical cancer, ovarian cancer, and cancers of the uterus. Pediatric oncologists treat cancer in children, and neurological oncologists treat brain tumors. Oncologists play a large role in preventative care. They emphasize the importance of sunscreen to avoid melanoma, they advise people against smoking to avoid lung, esophageal, or oral cancer. They warn against drinking liquor to avoid liver damage and cancer. Overall, oncologists play a vital role in helping cancer patients navigate the challenges that come with a cancer diagnosis, they provide medical expertise, and emotional support throughout the process.

Becoming an oncologist requires dedication and empathy, as they deal with patients facing challenging medical conditions. It begins with obtaining a bachelor's degree and fulfilling all the prerequisite courses for medical school in college or university. The prerequisite courses for medical school include physics, biology, chemistry, organic chemistry, and English classes. In order to attend medical school, students need to take the MCAT (Medical College Admissions Test). Most students typically take it in their third year of college or university. It's important to aim for a competitive score to gain acceptance into medical school. The MCAT is challenging, but it prepares students for medical school. Once accepted into medical school, it takes four years to complete. Medical school consists of 2 years of classroom study on subjects such as anatomy, biochemistry, and pharmacology, and the last 2 years consist of clinical rotations in several specialties, which may include oncology. Rotations during medical school can range from 4-8 weeks in length. An oncology rotation builds on a student's knowledge of general and surgical oncology, and sense of empathy. After medical school, students graduate with a degree in M.D. (Doctor of Medicine) or D.O. (Doctor of Osteopathic Medicine). The difference between the two is that MDs tend to take a more medication-focused approach to medicine, while DOs take a more holistic approach to medicine and focus on healing the whole body. Oncologists need to complete a three-year residency in internal medicine. Internal medicine is one of the less competitive residencies. During internal medicine residency, topics on oncology and cancer treatment are covered. In the years of medical school and residency, physicians will need to complete all three steps of the USMLE (United States Medical Licensing Examination) or COMLEX (Comprehensive Osteopathic Medical Licensing Exam). After the completion of residency, aspiring oncologists will need to apply for a 2-3 year oncology fellowship. During this fellowship, oncologists receive specialized training in oncology and gain exposure to various cancer treatment methods. Some oncologists choose to specialize even further and pursue a subspecialty like radiation oncology, surgical oncology, pediatric oncology, and more. After completing all their training, oncologists need to obtain a medical license and can choose to become board-certified. If they choose to become board-certified, they will need to pass an exam issued by the American Board of Internal Medicine (ABIM) or American Osteopathic Board of Internal Medicine (AOBIM). Oncology is a fulfilling specialty that allows physicians to make a significant impact on their patients by providing them with medical and emotional support throughout their journey.

Why You Should Become an Oncologist

Evolving

Oncology is a constantly evolving field with new discoveries and treatments

Patient Relationships

Oncologists develop strong bonds with their patients and care for them in a challenging part of their lives

Teamwork

Oncologists get to work with all kinds of doctors such as surgeons, radiologists, pathologists, and more.

Career Paths

There are many subspecialties in oncology, and oncologists can work in multiple settings

Oncology Trivia

1. What is the primary purpose of chemotherapy in cancer treatment?
    a. To surgically remove the tumor
    b. To boost the immune system
    c. To kill or slow the growth of cancer cells
    d. To reduce pain and discomfort

2. Which two cancers are often known as "silent killers" because their early-stage symptoms are usually not noticeable?
    a. Breast cancer, lung cancer
    b. Pancreatic cancer, ovarian cancer
    c. Skin cancer, uterine cancer
    d. Lung cancer, skin cancer

3. Which famous cyclist and cancer survivor started the Livestrong Foundation to support cancer patients and research?
    a. Lance Armstrong
    b. Micheal Phelps
    c. Usain Bolt
    d. Serena Williams

4. About how many people die a year from cancer?
    a. 20 million
    b. 5 million
    c. 10 million
    d. 13 million

All answers on next page

Oncology Trivia

1. What is the primary purpose of chemotherapy in cancer treatment?
    a. To surgically remove the tumor
    b. To boost the immune system
    c. To kill or slow the growth of cancer cells
    d. To reduce pain and discomfort

2. Which two cancers are often known as "silent killers" because their early-stage symptoms are usually not noticeable?
    a. Breast cancer, lung cancer
    b. Pancreatic cancer, ovarian cancer
    c. Skin cancer, uterine cancer
    d. Lung cancer, skin cancer

3. Which famous cyclist and cancer survivor started the Livestrong Foundation to support cancer patients and research?
    a. Lance Armstrong
    b. Micheal Phelps
    c. Usain Bolt
    d. Serena Williams

4. About how many people die from cancer each year?
    a. 20 million
    b. 5 million
    c. 10 million
    d. 13 million

Oncology Fun Facts

1. Being physically active can reduce the risks of developing colon, breast, and endometrial cancers

2. Cancer is the second-leading cause of death worldwide

3. The most common cancer is breast cancer

4. Heart cancer is extremely rare

5. World Cancer Day is on February 4th

6. The pink ribbon is the internationally recognized symbol for breast cancer awareness

7. Smoking causes about 20% of all cancers and about 30% of all cancer deaths in the U.S

Optometry & Ophthalmology

Optometry is a specialized field of healthcare that focuses on the examination, diagnosis, and treatment of various visual and ocular conditions. Optometrists are the primary healthcare professionals in this field and are referred to as Doctors of Optometry (OD). They are not medical doctors (MD) or doctors of osteopathy (DO). Optometrists diagnose and treat eye disease and vision problems. They can perform eye exams to determine the overall health of the eyes and prescribe corrective lenses, such as glasses or contact lenses to improve vision. Optometrists are trained to diagnose a wide range of eye conditions and visual disorders including nearsightedness, farsightedness, color blindness, cataracts (cloudiness on the eye's lens), astigmatism (part of the eye is more curved than it should be), presbyopia (loss of clear close-up vision), and more. Optometrists can prescribe medication for their patients who may be experiencing eye infections, inflammation, and other eye-related issues. Optometrists work closely with ophthalmologists and refer their patients to them if necessary. Ophthalmology is the medical specialty that focuses on the diagnosis and treatment of diseases, disorders, and injuries related to the eyes and visual system. Ophthalmologists are experts in the diagnosis and treatment of eye conditions. According to Cleveland Clinic, "An ophthalmologist is qualified to deliver total eye care, meaning eye examinations, medical and surgical care, and diagnosis and treatment of disease and visual complications that are caused by other conditions, like diabetes." Unlike optometrists, ophthalmologists are medical doctors (MD) or doctors of osteopathy (DO). They can conduct thorough eye exams and identify any vision or ocular issues. They have the ability to manage a range of eye diseases including but not limited to, cataracts, glaucoma (optic nerve damage from fluid buildup in the eye), and retinal detachment (retina pulls away from the tissues supporting it). Ophthalmologists are highly skilled in performing various surgical procedures and use surgery to correct these conditions. Other common procedures they may perform include cataract surgery, LASIK (Laser-assisted In Situ Keratomileusis) corneal transplants, retinal surgery, and many more. Similar to optometrists, ophthalmologists can prescribe medication and provide care to children. Ophthalmologists are trained to tend to eye injuries and emergencies, they can provide appropriate medical and surgical interventions. Nonetheless, both optometrists and ophthalmologists are healthcare professionals who undergo significant training to preserve and improve vision and overall eye health.

Becoming an optometrist requires a specific educational path and training. It begins with completing a bachelor's degree in a relevant field such as biology, chemistry, and physics. Maintaining a high GPA (Grade Point Average) and getting good grades are essential for optometry school. In order to apply for optometry school, students need to take the OAT (Optometry Admissions Test). This test is essential for optometry school and shows programs how prepared you are to begin learning the fundamentals of optometry. After being accepted into optometry school, it takes 4 years to earn a Doctor of Optometry degree (OD). During optometry school, students undergo training to learn about eye anatomy, ocular diseases, and vision-correcting techniques. Optometry school graduates have the option of completing a 1-year residency to gain more training and experience. After completing all of their training optometrists become board-certified by passing an exam issued by the NBEO (National Board of Examiners in Optometry), and obtain a license to begin practicing optometry. Becoming an optometrist is quite different than becoming an ophthalmologist. Becoming an ophthalmologist requires much more training compared to optometrists. They begin with obtaining a bachelor's degree while fulfilling the prerequisite courses for medical school. In order to apply to medical school, students need to take the MCAT (Medical College Admissions Test). A high MCAT score is crucial to gain acceptance into medical school. During medical school, students complete clinical rotations in several specialties, which may include ophthalmology. Also during medical school, students take the first parts of the USMLE (United States Medical Licensing Examination) or COMLEX (Comprehensive Osteopathic Licensing Examination). Once a student has gained a passion for ophthalmology, they can begin thinking about applying for ophthalmology residency. Ophthalmology residency is three years in length, during the first year of their residency, residents are known as interns. During residency, residents gain hands-on experience and become experts in eye care and eye surgery. Following the completion of their residency, ophthalmologists can consider pursuing a fellowship, becoming board-certified, and obtaining a license. Some ophthalmologic fellowships include cornea and refractive surgery, pediatric ophthalmology, vitreoretinal surgery, neuro-ophthalmology, and more. Board certification is not mandatory, but it demonstrates a physician's expertise and dedication to their field. To begin practicing medicine, a physician needs to be licensed in their state. The path to becoming an optometrist and ophthalmologist is lengthy but the reward is a fulfilling career focused on the diagnosis and treatment of eye diseases and conditions.

Why You Should Become an Optometrist or Ophthalmologist

Quality of life

Vision is a valuable sense, optometrists and ophthalmologists can improve someone's quality of life

Work-life balance

Most ophthalmologists find balance in their career and are satisfied with their specialty

Technology

Ophthalmologists can work with lasers, microscopes, cameras, and other tools

Patient settings

Optometrists can work in retail locations, clinics, and hospitals

Optometry & Ophthalmology Trivia

1. What is the medical term for "pink eye"?

    a. Conjunctivitis

    b. Hyperopia

    c. Edema

    d. Cataracts

2. What is the part of the eye that helps produce tears to keep the eyes moist?

    a. The sclera

    b. The optic nerve

    c. The lacrimal gland

    d. The choroid

3. When is World Sight Day?

    a. February 12

    b. April 15

    c. October 12

    d. October 18

4. What is the medical term for nearsightedness?

    a. Nearbyopoia

    b. Laserscelorosis

    c. Myopia

    d. Retinitis

Answers on next page

Optometry & Ophthalmology Trivia

1. What is the medical term for "pink eye"?

    a. Conjunctivitis

    b. Hyperopia

    c. Edema

    d. Cataracts

2. What is the part of the eye that helps produce tears to keep the eyes moist?

    a. The sclera

    b. The optic nerve

    c. The lacrimal gland

    d. The choroid

3. When is World Sight Day?

    a. February 12

    b. April 15

    c. October 12

    d. October 18

4. What is the medical term for nearsightedness?

    a. Nearbyopoia

    b. Lasersclerosis

    c. Myopia

    d. Retinitis

Optometry & Ophthalmology Fun Facts

1. The human eye can detect about 10 million different colors

2. On average, the human eye blinks 15-20 times per minute, which is around 1200 times an hour

3. The first corneal transplant was performed in 1905

4. The retina contains about 91 million rod cells and about 4.5 million cones

5. More than 75% of U.S adults need some form of vision correction, either glasses or contact lenses

6. Some animals have better vision than humans, eagles and cheetahs can see miles away

Orthopedics

Orthopedics is the medical specialty that focuses on the diagnosis and treatment of disorders related to the musculoskeletal system. The musculoskeletal system is made up of bones, ligaments, tendons, and cartilage. Orthopedic doctors, also known as orthopedic surgeons are medical professionals who specialize in this field. They are trained to provide both surgical and non-surgical treatments for various musculoskeletal injuries and conditions. Orthopedic surgeons can manage fractures and dislocations, they can set broken bones and repair dislocated joints. They discuss treatment options and meet with their patients throughout their healing process. Orthopedic surgeons are very familiar with sports injuries, such as ligament tears, tendon injuries, and fractures. They are also familiar with various types of arthritis. This includes osteoarthritis, rheumatoid arthritis, and juvenile arthritis. Rheumatologists are also experts in treating these types of conditions. Orthopedic surgeons perform joint replacement surgeries, such as knee replacement, hip replacement, and shoulder replacement. These surgeries are typically done to relieve pain and improve joint function in patients. Both neurosurgeons and orthopedic surgeons are skilled in performing surgery on the spine. An orthopedic surgeon can address spine-related issues like scoliosis, herniated discs, and spinal stenosis (when the space inside the backbone is too small).They also play a large role in trauma cases. They can manage injuries resulting from accidents or traumatic events, often involving multiple fractures, bones, and complex injuries. Orthopedic surgeons can treat congenital deformities, they can treat children who have musculoskeletal abnormalities and developmental disorders. Some congenital deformities they may treat include clubfoot and hip dysplasia. In order to diagnose and treat the abnormalities, conditions, and diseases listed above, orthopedic specialists use several diagnostic tools. They can use a combination of X-rays, MRIs, CT scans, and physical examinations to evaluate their patients' conditions accurately. Based on their findings, they design individualized treatment plans that may involve medications, surgery, braces, casts, physical therapy, and more to help their patients. The differences between orthopedic physicians and rheumatologists are often unclear. A rheumatologist can treat many of the same conditions as orthopedic surgeons. Rheumatologists do not perform surgery, and receive training in rheumatic disease. Orthopedic surgeons play a crucial role in helping people recover from musculoskeletal injuries and conditions, restore their mobility, reduce pain, and enhance their quality of life.

Becoming an orthopedic surgeon requires a significant dedication to education, training, and professional development. All physicians need to begin by obtaining a bachelor's degree and fulfilling the prerequisite courses for medical school. Students typically take classes such as biology, chemistry, organic chemistry, biochemistry, and genetics to prepare for medical school. Students typically take the MCAT (Medical College Admissions Test) in their third year of college or university. A high MCAT score along with a strong GPA (Grade Point Average) is essential for gaining acceptance into medical school. Other important factors for acceptance into medical school are research projects, clinical experience, recommendation letters, and volunteer hours. Once accepted into medical school it will take four years to complete. During medical school, students complete clinical rotations in different specialties, including orthopedic surgery. It is during this time that students hope to find a passion for a medical specialty and soon apply for residency. During the fourth year of medical school, students begin applying for residency. Orthopedic surgery is a competitive field, in 2022 about 40% of applicants did not successfully match. Throughout medical school and the first year of residency, physicians must complete all three steps of the USMLE (United States Medical Licensing Examination) or COMLEX (Comprehensive Osteopathic Medical Licensing Exam). During residency, residents learn to perform clinical procedures, write prescriptions, and learn the fundamentals of orthopedic surgery. After graduating from residency, orthopedic surgeons can consider pursuing a fellowship. Some orthopedic surgery fellowships include orthopedic trauma, pediatric orthopedics, sports medicine, and more. They also have the option of becoming board-certified, which demonstrates a physician's expertise in their field. Board-certification is obtained by passing an exam issued by the American Board of Orthopedic Surgery. Lastly, to begin practicing medicine in their location, a physician needs to obtain a license. The journey to becoming an orthopedic surgeon is lengthy and challenging but is also extremely rewarding.

Why You Should Become an Orthopedic Surgeon

Patient Impact

Orthopedic surgeons can improve their patient's mobility, reduce their pain, and help them regain their independence

Respected Profession

Orthopedic surgeons are highly respected and are experts in their field

High Salary

An orthopedic surgeon can make up to $754,850 in the U.S

Job Security

Orthopedic surgeons are always in demand

Orthopedics Trivia

1. Which surgical procedure involves replacing a damaged joint with an artificial one, often made of metal and plastic?
    a. Scoliosis correction surgery
    b. ACL reconstruction surgery
    c. Joint replacement surgery
    d. Joint fusion

2. Which anatomical structure separates the thigh from the lower leg and is often called the "shin bone"?
    a. The Femur
    b. The Patella
    c. The Tibia
    d. The Fibula

3. Which type of fracture involves the bone breaking into multiple fragments?
    a. Comminuted fracture
    b. Stable fracture
    c. Transverse fracture
    d. Open fracture

4. What is the term for the condition in which a part of the bone dies due to a lack of blood supply?
    a. Fibromyalgia
    b. Kyphosis
    c. Avascular necrosis
    d. Osteoarthritis

All answers on next page

Orthopedics Trivia

1. Which surgical procedure involves replacing a damaged joint with an artificial one, often made of metal and plastic?
    a. Scoliosis correction surgery
    b. ACL reconstruction surgery
    c. Joint replacement surgery
    d. Joint fusion

2. Which anatomical structure separates the thigh from the lower leg and is often called the "shin bone"?
    a. The Femur
    b. The Patella
    c. The Tibia
    d. The fibula

3. Which type of fracture involves the bone breaking into multiple fragments?
    a. Comminuted fracture
    b. Stable fracture
    c. Transverse fracture
    d. Open fracture

4. What is the term for the condition in which a part of the bone dies due to a lack of blood supply?
    a. Fibromyalgia
    b. Kyphosis
    c. Avascular necrosis
    d. Osteoarthritis

Orthopedics Fun Facts

1. October is Bone and Joint Health Awareness Month

2. Bones can repair themselves after a minor break or fracture

3. Dr. Robert Malt and his team performed the first successful reattachment of a severed limb

4. Over 450,000 hip replacements are performed annually in the U.S

5. The most common form of arthritis is osteoarthritis

6. Arthritis is the leading cause of work disability in the U.S

Pathology

Pathology is the medical specialty that is defined as the science of the causes and effects of diseases, it especially deals with the laboratory examination of tissue samples for diagnostic or forensic purposes. Pathologists are medical doctors who specialize in pathology and examine tissues, organs, and bodily fluids to determine the cause and nature of diseases. They can perform a wide range of tasks. Pathologists examine biopsies and fluids collected from patients to identify the presence of diseases such as cancer, infections, autoimmune disorders, and genetic conditions. Using this information, they can provide insight and information on how to diagnose and treat conditions. According to the Cleveland Clinic, "pathologists can work in all areas of medicine, such as oncology, immunology, and genetics." They also work closely with other medical specialists like radiologists, surgeons, oncologists, and more. The main role of pathologists is to perform lab tests which include pap smears, biopsies, blood sugar tests, and autopsies. An autopsy is a medical exam of a body after death. Forensic pathologists are responsible for performing autopsies in the case of sudden, unexpected, or suspicious deaths. Pathologists analyze autopsy results and medical history to determine if a death was natural, accidental, or by another cause. There are several types of pathologists. Dermatopathologists interpret skin biopsies and help diagnose skin diseases. Neuropathologists help diagnose neurological diseases. Pediatric pathology is the study of pathology in children, and cytopathologists help diagnose cancer. Pathologists are involved in grading tumors or cancer and participate in their staging in order to estimate tumor and cancer progression (more details in the chapter on Oncology). Pathologists also oversee laboratories and ensure that lab tests and results are accurate and reliable. They can help develop and validate new laboratory tests. Unlike other physicians, pathologists don't usually interact with patients. They play a large role in determining the diagnosis, but another physician often tells the patient about their diagnosis. Despite not interacting with patients, pathologists play a tremendous part in medical research. They contribute to medical advancements by studying the cellular and molecular basis of diseases. "They work to develop new treatments to fight or prevent viruses, infections and diseases." The Royal College of Pathologists says that pathology "is the bridge between science and medicine." Pathologists play a vital role in healthcare by providing essential information for patient care and advancing the world's understanding of illness and disease.

The general steps to becoming a pathologist require 11-12 years of training and specialization after high school. It begins with completing a bachelor's degree while fulfilling the prerequisite courses for medical school. Prerequisite courses for medical school include physics, biology, chemistry, biochemistry, organic chemistry, and English classes. Helpful courses for medical school also include genetics, histology, and human physiology. Students typically take the MCAT (Medical College Admissions Test) in their third year of college or university. The MCAT is a challenging exam that requires a competitive score for entrance into medical school. After obtaining a bachelor's degree and taking the MCAT, aspiring pathologists need to attend medical school to become a Medical Doctor (MD) or Doctor of Osteopathic Medicine (DO). M.D. programs typically have a very slim acceptance rate, while D.O. programs often have a higher acceptance rate. During medical school, students take the first parts of the USMLE (United States Medical Licensing Examination) or COMLEX (Comprehensive Osteopathic Medical Licensing Exam). In their final years of medical school, students begin to prepare for residency. This process involves determining which specialty they are most passionate about, and applying for residency. Pathology residency is 3-4 years long. The third step of the USMLE or COMLEX is commonly taken during the first year of residency. During residency, residents receive specialized training in anatomical or clinical pathology, which covers a wide range of laboratory testing, diagnostics, and disease analysis. After the completion of their residency, pathologists may consider pursuing a fellowship. Pathology fellowships include but are not limited to, cytopathology, dermatopathology, gastrointestinal pathology, breast pathology, and surgical pathology, which were discussed above. These fellowships are commonly 1-2 years long. Once all of their training is complete pathologists have the option to become board certified. Becoming board-certified in pathology requires passing an examination issued by the American Board of Pathology. The clinical pathology examination includes 330 questions, and the entirety of the exam is about 6 and ½ hours in length. Lastly, in order to begin practicing medicine, a physician needs to obtain a license. When training to become a pathologist, it's important to have a genuine interest in medical science, and disease analysis. Pathologists play a critical role in healthcare, research, and patient diagnoses

Why You Should Become a Pathologist

Intellectually Stimulating

Pathologists use problem-solving skills to study and investigate the cause and nature of diseases every day

Technology

Pathologists use cutting-edge laboratory techniques, analyze bodily fluids, and conduct research

Lab Experts

Pathologists are well-versed with all sorts of tests, procedures, imaging techniques, and infections

High Salary

The College of American Pathologists reports that the average pathologist makes $308,000 annually

Pathology Trivia

1. Which cells in the blood are responsible for fighting infections?
    a. Platelets
    b. White blood cells
    c. Red blood cells
    d. Cancer cells

2. Which types of cells are responsible for producing antibodies in response to infections?
    a. T cells
    b. White blood cells
    c. B cells
    d. Neurons

3. How many basic types of tissue are there?
    a. 3
    b. 8
    c. 11
    d. 4

4. A pathologist would typically **not** perform a?
    a. Stress test
    b. Blood test
    c. Cancer screening
    d. Autopsy

All answers on next page

Pathology Trivia

1. Which cells in the blood are responsible for fighting infections?

    a. Platelets

    b. White blood cells

    c. Red blood cells

    d. Cancer cells

2. Which types of cells are responsible for producing antibodies in response to infections?

    a. T cells

    b. White blood cells

    c. B cells

    d. Neurons

3. How many basic types of tissue are there?

    a. 3

    b. 8

    c. 11

    d. 4

4. A pathologist would typically **not** perform a?

    a. Stress test

    b. Blood test

    c. Cancer screening

    d. Autopsy

Pathology Fun Facts

1. Humans have 20,000-25,000 genes

2. Robert Hooke discovered cells using a compound microscope

3. Pathologists can work in several locations like hospitals, clinics, laboratories, and other medical facilities

4. Pathology is not an overly competitive field

5. More than 60% of the human body is made up of water, every part of the body needs water

6. Sweat is almost completely made up of water

7. The human body makes about 3-8 cups of urine every day

Pediatrics

Pediatrics is the branch of medicine that focuses on the medical care of infants, children, and adolescents. Pediatricians are medical doctors who specialize in the health and well-being of young individuals, from birth through adolescence. Pediatricians are trained to diagnose, treat, and prevent a wide range of medical conditions and illnesses that are specific to this age group. They ensure the overall health of children and have several responsibilities. A pediatrician performs wellness checkups, which are regular checkups that monitor the growth, development, and overall health of a child. They often take note of the child's height, weight, hearing, vision, heartbeat, and posture. Pediatricians can diagnose and treat many health conditions, illnesses, and injuries. This ranges from strep throat to much more complex issues such as chronic diseases, and genetic disorders. Other issues they often see in children include asthma, diabetes, and allergies. In order to deal with these conditions and illnesses, a pediatrician will prescribe medication. Pediatricians also administer and encourage vaccines to protect their young patients from various diseases and help establish immunity. Some common vaccinations a pediatrician may administer are the hepatitis B vaccine, the HPV vaccine, flu vaccines, the MMR vaccine, and more. Pediatricians address behavioral and developmental disorders. They may catch these disorders in their patients and diagnose them with ADHD (Attention deficit hyperactivity disorder), autism spectrum disorder, a learning disability, or another. Pediatricians are also mental health advocates. They can help their patients who may be struggling with their mental health, give them advice, and counsel their patients. Pediatricians commonly advise their young patients to eat a healthy diet, be physically active, and get at least 8 hours of sleep every night. Pediatricians also listen to parents' concerns and answer any questions they may have. There are several kinds of tests a pediatrician may perform or order. These include newborn screening tests, hearing tests, STD screenings, sports physicals, and mental health screenings. If it is necessary, a pediatrician may refer their patient to another specialist for further evaluation. They may refer them to a cardiologist if their patient has a heart murmur, or they might refer them to an orthopedic surgeon to treat their scoliosis. The world of pediatrics is not only limited to pediatricians. There are pediatric surgeons, pediatric cardiologists, pediatric neurosurgeons, pediatric oncologists, and more. These specialists and pediatricians help to promote the health and well-being of infants, children, and adolescents ensuring they have a healthy future.

Becoming a pediatrician begins with completing a bachelor's degree while fulfilling all the prerequisite courses for medical school. These include English, chemistry, organic chemistry, biology, biochemistry, and physics classes. Students typically take the MCAT (Medical College Admissions Test) in their third year of college or university. The MCAT ranges from the lowest score being a 472 and the highest possible score being a 528. It is a great factor in being accepted into medical school. Once accepted into medical school the first two years consist of lectures, and a range of subjects such as anatomy, physiology, pharmacology, and more. During medical school, students often take the first parts of the USMLE (United States Medical Licensing Exam) or COMLEX (Comprehensive Osteopathic Medical Licensing Exam). Also during medical school, students complete clinical rotations in several medical specialties, which may include pediatrics. During the final year of medical school, students hope to match into residency. Pediatric residency has a high match rate, and it is considered an averagely competitive specialty. A pediatric residency program lasts three years. During their residency, pediatricians become experts in the care of infants, children, and adolescents. Residents will work under the guidance of experienced pediatricians, gain hands-on experience, and are trained to diagnose and treat a wide range of conditions. Following the completion of residency, pediatricians have the option to complete a fellowship. The most popular pediatric fellowships include pediatric cardiology, pediatric emergency medicine, pediatric endocrinology, pediatric oncology, and more. These fellowships are not mandatory but are 2-3 years in length. Pediatricians can also consider becoming board-certified by passing an exam issued by the The American Board of Pediatrics. Becoming board-certified demonstrates a physician's expertise and dedication to their field. The exam is about 7 hours long, it deeply tests doctors on their knowledge in the field of pediatrics. After completing all their training, a pediatrician must obtain a license to begin practicing medicine in their location. Pediatricians along with all other medical specialties must stay up to date with the latest medical advancements, research, and technology. Overall, becoming a pediatrician requires hard work and a passion for working with children and their families. Pediatrics allows physicians to make a positive impact on the lives of their young patients and their communities.

Why You Should Become a Pediatrician

Working with Children

People who enjoy working with children and babies should definitely look into pediatrics

Variety

There are several specialties to work in pediatrics such as orthopedics, cardiology, neurology, oncology, and more

Job satisfaction

Working with children is fun, pediatrics is less tense than other specialties

Continuity of care

Pediatricians work with their patients from birth till the age of 21

Pediatrics Trivia

1. Which disorder involves the immune system attacking and damaging the small intestine in response to gluten consumption?
    a. Hydrocephalus
    b. Celiac disease
    c. Lactose intolerance
    d. Bronchitis

2. What is the name for a severe, life-threatening allergic reaction that can develop rapidly?
    a. Anaphylaxis
    b. Epinephrine
    c. Asthma
    d. Influenza

3. ____ occurs when a baby's bilirubin levels become elevated, causing yellowing of the skin and eyes
    a. Colic
    b. Hydronephrosis
    c. Jaundice
    d. Apnea

4. Fifth disease is common in children, what is another name for it?
    a. Slapped cheek syndrome
    b. Rosacea
    c. Baby blushing syndrome
    d. Severe eczema

All answers on next page

Pediatrics Trivia

1. What childhood disorder involves the immune system attacking and damaging the small intestine in response to gluten consumption?
    a. Hydrocephalus
    b. Celiac disease
    c. Lactose intolerance
    d. Bronchitis

2. What is the name for a severe, life-threatening allergic reaction that can develop rapidly?
    a. Anaphylaxis
    b. Epinephrine
    c. Asthma
    d. Influenza

3. ___ occurs when a baby's bilirubin levels become elevated, causing yellowing of the skin and eyes
    a. Colic
    b. Hydronephrosis
    c. Jaundice
    d. Apnea

4. Fifth disease is common in children, what is another name for it?
    a. Slapped cheek syndrome
    b. Rosacea
    c. Baby blushing syndrome
    d. Severe eczema

Pediatrics Fun Facts

1. Pediatricians wear colored stethoscopes, scrubs, and use toys during examinations to make their young patients feel comfortable and relaxed

2. Abraham Jacobi is known as "the father of American pediatrics"

3. Children have 20 teeth, once they fall out, they will typically have 32 adult teeth

4. Most young infants need to eat 100-120 calories a day

5. Research suggests that children who nurse for 6+ months are less likely to have childhood leukemia and lymphoma

Plastic surgery

Plastic surgery is the medical specialty that deals with the repair, reconstruction, and alteration of the human body's appearance and function. The term 'plastics' is derived from the Greek word "plastikos" which means to form or mold, it is not the actual use of plastic during surgery. Plastic surgeons can repair injuries, congenital defects, and use cosmetic procedures to enhance or alter someone's features. Some of the most common cosmetic surgeries a plastic surgeon performs are breast augmentations, liposuctions, rhinoplasties (nose jobs), and facelifts. These surgeries focus on enhancing a person's appearance to often achieve a certain look or reverse the effects of aging. Other cosmetic procedures they may perform are botox injections, brow lifts, and hair transplantations. Hair transplants are minimally invasive procedures that are used in areas of balding, to restore eyelashes, eyebrows, and more. These procedures are typically elective and are chosen by individuals who want to improve their features. Plastic surgeons are experts in repairing birth defects affecting someone's appearance or function. They may operate on cleft lip and palate, syndactyly (webbed fingers or toes), microtia (abnormality of the outer ear), and more. Plastic surgeons use several techniques to treat severe injuries and to restore a person's appearance after experiencing trauma. They can perform skin grafts which is when a plastic surgeon removes a piece of healthy skin and attaches it to a different part of the body, these can help treat burn wounds. They also use techniques to help with complex wounds, lacerations, facial injuries, and scarring. A plastic surgeon also has the ability to reattach a limb or part of the body that has been severed. Plastic surgeons play a large role in jaw surgery as the jaw is actually a delicate part of the human body. They are qualified to perform jaw surgery which can improve a patient's breathing and overall appearance. Did you know that nearly 450,000 people suffer from burn injuries in the United States each year? According to the American Society of Plastic Surgeons, "plastic surgeons are integral to the care of both pediatric and adult patients suffering from burn injuries." Plastic surgeons can manage complex burns and use methods such as skin grafts, flaps, and free tissue transfers to treat them. In summary, plastic surgery involves a range of procedures and surgeries aimed at restoring, reconstructing, and enhancing the appearance and function of different parts of the body. Plastic surgeons have expertise in both reconstruction and aesthetic aspects of surgery and play a vital role in improving patients' physical well-being and self-esteem.

Becoming a plastic surgeon involves several years of education and training. It begins with earning a bachelor's degree and fulfilling the prerequisite courses for medical school. These include English, biology, chemistry, organic chemistry, and physics classes. Students typically take the MCAT (Medical College Admissions Test) in their third year of college or university. The MCAT is a challenging exam that can take several months to prepare for, yet a high score is crucial for acceptance into medical school. An outstanding medical school application includes clinical experience, a high MCAT score, volunteer hours, a high GPA (Grade Point Average), and research projects. Once accepted into medical school, it takes four years to earn a Doctor of Medicine (MD) or Doctor of Osteopathic Medicine (DO) degree. The first two years of medical school consist of classroom learning, lectures, and covering subjects such as anatomy, physiology, pharmacology, and biochemistry. The last two years of medical school consist of clinical rotations in several medical specialties and applying for residency. Plastic surgery residency is one of the most competitive residencies to match into. There are two main ways to complete a residency in plastic surgery. Aspiring plastic surgeons can complete a 6-year plastic surgery residency which deeply covers reconstructive and cosmetic surgery. The other route is to complete a residency in general, or ear nose and throat surgery, and then get training in plastic surgery. Both residency routes instill plastic surgeons with the fundamentals of plastic surgery, cosmetic surgery, and reconstructive surgery. During residency, plastic surgeons have the opportunity to work with experienced surgeons and gain hands-on experience in the operating room. Throughout medical school and residency, physicians will have to complete all parts of the USMLE (United States Medical Licensing Exam) or COMLEX (Comprehensive Osteopathic Medical Licensing Exam). After the completion of residency, plastic surgeons can consider pursuing a fellowship. Subspecialties within plastic surgery include craniofacial surgery, hand surgery, burn surgery, otoplasty, and more. These fellowships require an extra 1-2 years of training. Plastic surgeons can become board-certified by passing an exam by the American Board of Plastic Surgery. Board certification is not mandatory but it demonstrates a physician's expertise and dedication to their field. After completing all of their training, plastic surgeons need to obtain a license to begin practicing medicine in their location. Plastic surgeons can work in private practices, hospitals, and surgery centers. It is important to note that becoming a plastic surgeon is demanding and competitive. Plastic surgery is an extremely rewarding field but it demands a high level of education, and the ability to handle complex surgical procedures.

Why You Should Become a Plastic Surgeon

Combination of Art and Science

Plastic surgery combines science with artistic skill

High Salary

The salary of plastic surgeons ranges, but they can make up to $690,000 a year

Job Satisfaction

Plastic surgeons have the ability to increase someone's self-esteem and confidence

Technology

Plastic surgeons work with cutting-edge surgical techniques, and plastic surgery is an evolving field

Plastic Surgery Trivia

1. Which ancient surgeon is known as the originator of plastic surgery?
    a. J. Marion Sims
    b. Johann Reil
    c. Shushruta
    d. Daniel Coit Gilman

2. What is the medical term for breast reduction surgery, often performed by plastic surgeons?
    a. Mammogram
    b. Mastectomy
    c. Reduction mammoplasty
    d. Reduction mastectomy

3. What is the term for the process of transferring tissue from one part of the body to the other, often used in reconstructive surgery?
    a. Tissue graft
    b. Tissue transplantation
    c. Rhinoplasty
    d. Tisoscopy

4. What is the term for the surgical procedure that changes the shape, size, or position of the ears?
    a. Otoplasty
    b. Ptosis
    c. Blepharoplasty
    d. Brachioplasty

All answers on next page

Plastic Surgery Trivia

1. Which ancient surgeon is known as the originator of plastic surgery?
    a. J. Marion Sims
    b. Johann Reil
    c. Shushruta
    d. Daniel Coit Gilman

2. What is the medical term for breast reduction surgery, often performed by plastic surgeons?
    a. Mammogram
    b. Mastectomy
    c. Reduction mammoplasty
    d. Reduction mastectomy

3. What is the term for the process of transferring tissue from one part of the body to the other, often used in reconstructive surgery?
    a. Tissue graft
    b. Tissue transplantation
    c. Rhinoplasty
    d. Tisoscopy

4. What is the term for the surgical procedure that changes the shape, size, or position of the ears?
    a. Otoplasty
    b. Ptosis
    c. Blepharoplasty
    d. Brachioplasty

Plastic Surgery Fun Facts

1. Plastic surgery has two main branches, cosmetic and reconstructive

2. The most common plastic surgery nationwide is breast augmentation

3. Americans spent more than $16.5 billion on cosmetic plastic surgery in 2018

4. Plastic surgery was common during the world wars to help soldiers who had deformities after battle

5. Plastic surgery addiction is a harmful condition that can affect people with body dysmorphic disorder

Psychiatry

Psychiatry is the branch of medicine that focuses on the diagnosis, treatment, and prevention of mental illnesses and disorders. Psychiatry is a dynamic field that continues to contribute significantly to the world's understanding of the human mind and the treatment of mental health disorders. Psychiatrists are medical doctors who specialize in mental health care and are trained to understand all the factors that contribute to mental health and well-being. The ultimate goal of psychiatrists is to help their patients achieve better mental health and improve their quality of life. People may need to see a psychiatrist for many different reasons. Psychiatrists are trained to recognize various mental health disorders through careful assessment, patient interviews, behavior patterns, symptoms, and medical history. These evaluations help paint a picture of their patient's mental well-being. Once they have made a diagnosis, they can begin discussing treatment plans with their patient. Psychiatrists can use a variety of treatments. Psychotherapy is also known as talk therapy, this is when the patient discusses their symptoms or troubles, hoping to eliminate them. Yet, every patient is different and psychiatrists may work with them for a few weeks, months, or even years to solve their mental issues. Psychiatrists may also prescribe medication to aid their patients. Antidepressants are used to treat depression, sedatives are used to treat insomnia and anxiety, and stimulants are used to treat ADHD (Attention Deficit Hyperactivity Disorder). These medications are known to reduce the symptoms of psychiatric disorders. In cases of severe depression that does not respond to other treatments, a psychiatrist may use electroconvulsive therapy (ECT) which applies electrical currents to the brain. Other new treatments in psychiatry involve deep brain stimulation (DBS) and vagus nerve stimulation (VNS) to treat mental health disorders. Many psychiatrists engage in research to advance the world's understanding of mental health disorders and their underlying causes. Psychiatrists also play a role in public health by advocating for mental health awareness, education, and stigma reduction. They provide guidance on maintaining good health and preventing the onset of mental health disorders. Psychiatrists could arguably have the widest span of workplaces. They may work in private practices, hospitals, psychiatric hospitals, nursing homes, prisons, and more. While they have a broad span of workplaces, they also collaborate with other specialists. They may introduce their patients to psychologists and therapists. Psychiatry improves the lives of individuals affected by mental health conditions and promotes overall well-being.

Becoming a psychiatrist involves a comprehensive educational and training path. It begins with completing a bachelor's degree in a relevant field. Most students who want to go into psychiatry pursue a major in psychology, biology, neuroscience, chemistry, or another. Students typically take the MCAT (Medical College Admissions Test) in their third year of college or university. A high MCAT score is needed to gain acceptance into medical school. The scoring of the MCAT ranges from the lowest score being a 472 and the highest being 528. A well-rounded application for medical school includes clinical experience, volunteer hours, research projects, a high MCAT score, and excellent recommendation letters. Once they are accepted into medical school, they need to complete four years, and earn either a Doctor of Medicine (MD) or Doctor of Osteopathic Medicine (DO) degree. MDs are known to take more of a medication-focused approach to medicine, while DOs take a more holistic approach to medicine. During medical school, students take foundational medical courses, engage in clinical rotations, and gain exposure to several medical specialties. During the third and fourth years of medical school, students begin thinking about what specialty they are most interested in and apply for residency. Residency is the opportunity for physicians to specialize in their field and become experts in it. The overall competitiveness for matching into psychiatry is relatively low. Psychiatry residency is 4 years long. During their residency, psychiatrists gain hands-on experience in diagnosing and treating various mental health conditions. Upon the completion of their residency, psychiatrists can become board-certified and consider pursuing a fellowship. Board certification is not mandatory but becoming board certified requires passing an exam issued by the American Board of Psychiatry and Neurology. There are about 9 subspecialties within psychiatry, and they are each about 1-year in length. These include addiction psychiatry, geriatric psychiatry, forensic psychiatry, child and adolescent psychiatry, and more. After the completion of all their training and education, a physician must obtain a license to begin practicing medicine in their location. There are various settings where a psychiatrist can work such as general hospitals, psychiatric hospitals, prisons, nursing homes, private practices, and more. Becoming a psychiatrist requires a genuine interest in helping individuals with mental health issues. The journey is lengthy, but it is a rewarding path for those who are passionate about improving mental health and making a positive impact on people's lives.

Why You Should Become a Psychiatrist

Job Outlook

The job outlook for psychiatrists is expected to grow in the coming years

Added Skills

Becoming a psychiatrist means improving on communication, listening, and having empathy for others

Interesting work

Psychiatrists get to work with the brain, mental health disorders, and many types of patients

High Salary

Psychiatrists can make up to $250,000+

Psychiatry Trivia

1. Which neurotransmitter plays a role in many important body functions including memory, pleasurable reward, and motivation?
    a. Melatonin
    b. Cerebrum
    c. Dopamine
    d. Serorotin

2. What is the term for a mental disorder characterized by hallucinations, delusions, difficulty in social relationships, and reduced expression of emotions?
    a. Schizophrenia
    b. Bipolar Disorder
    c. ADHD
    d. Repression

3. Which part of the brain is often referred to as the "fight or flight" center and plays a role in memory?
    a. Frontal lobe
    b. Amygdala
    c. Broca's area
    d. The brain stem

4. What is the disorder characterized by sudden episodes of intense fear, discomfort, or a sense of losing control?
    a. OCD
    b. Panic disorder
    c. Eating disorder
    d. Mood disorder

All answers on next page

Psychiatry Trivia

1. Which neurotransmitter plays a role in many important body functions including memory, pleasurable reward, and motivation?
    a. Melatonin
    b. Cerebrum
    c. Dopamine
    d. Serotonin

2. What is the term for a mental disorder characterized by hallucinations, delusions, difficulty in social relationships, and reduced expression of emotions?
    a. Schizophrenia
    b. Bipolar disorder
    c. ADHD
    d. Repression

3. Which part of the brain is referred to as the "fight or flight" center and plays a role in memory?
    a. Frontal lobe
    b. Amygdala
    c. Broca's area
    d. The brain stem

4. What is the disorder characterized by sudden episodes of intense fear, discomfort, or a sense of losing control?
    a. OCD
    b. Panic disorder
    c. Eating disorder
    d. Mood disorder

Psychiatry Fun Facts

1. The Rorschach test, a famous psychological assessment uses inkblots to analyze a person's perceptions and emotions

2. The placebo effect is when a patient experiences improvement in symptoms after receiving a non-active treatment, it highlights the power of the mind in influencing physical well-being

3. The famous composer Wolfgang Mozart was known to suffer from depression

4. Laughter is great for mental health, it releases endorphins, which are the body's natural feel-good chemicals

5. Circadian rhythm is the body's "internal clock"

Radiology

Radiology is the medical specialty that involves the use of various imaging techniques to diagnose and treat conditions within the human body. Radiologists are medical doctors who specialize in interpreting medical images. They are trained to use and understand X-rays, CT (computerized tomography) scans, MRIs (magnetic resonance imaging), nuclear medicine scans, PET scans (positron emission tomography), and ultrasounds. X-rays use electromagnetic energy beams to produce images of bones, organs, and some soft tissues. CT scans are a combination of X-rays and computer technology to show incredibly detailed images of any part of the body. CT scans can show bones, organs, muscles, fat, blood vessels, internal injuries, and more. MRIs use a large magnet, radio waves, and a computer to show clear pictures of the brain, spinal cord, nerves, muscles, and ligaments. MRIs are typically much more expensive than CT scans. An ultrasound uses high-frequency sound waves to produce an image of internal structures. Ultrasounds are commonly used to examine developing fetuses in the uterus, someone's abdomen and pelvis, blood vessels, and more. According to the Cleveland Clinic, "PET scans detect early stages of cancer, heart disease, and brain conditions." These imaging tests play a crucial role in healthcare by providing insight into the internal structures of the body without the need for surgery. The role of radiologists is to interpret medical images to diagnose various conditions including fractures, tumors, infections, and abnormalities in organs. Radiologists assist in planning treatments, like surgery or radiation therapy, by providing detailed images that help other physicians target specific areas in the body. There are several types of radiologists. Diagnostic radiologists use a variety of imaging scans to assess a patient's condition. They direct radiology technicians, interpret and report their findings, and if necessary complete more imaging scans. According to the American College of Radiologists, "Interventional radiologists are doctors who diagnose and treat patients using image-guided, minimally invasive techniques such as X-rays and MRI." They use instruments through small incisions in the body to treat conditions without traditional surgery. Radiation oncologists oversee cancer patients' treatment plans and use radiation therapy to treat cancer. Radiologists are specialized doctors who play a vital role in making diagnoses, guiding medical procedures, and contributing to advancements in medical imaging technology. Radiology is a critical medical specialty that uses cutting-edge technology to diagnose and treat many medical conditions.

Becoming a radiologist is a journey that blends medical expertise with specialized training in diagnostic imaging techniques. It begins with obtaining a bachelor's degree in college or university. It is important to fulfill all the prerequisite courses for medical school and to prepare for the MCAT (Medical College Admissions Test). The MCAT is a challenging exam which most students take in their third year of college or university. A high MCAT score is essential for acceptance into medical school. An excellent application for medical school includes clinical experience, volunteer hours, research projects, recommendations from professors and peers, and a high MCAT score. After completing a bachelor's degree aspiring radiologists need to attend medical school to earn a Doctor of Medicine (MD) or Doctor of Osteopathic Medicine (DO) degree. The difference between the two is that MDs take a more medication-focused approach to medicine while DOs take a more holistic approach to medicine. During medical school, students complete clinical rotations in several medical specialties. They may rotate through internal medicine, OB/GYN, neurology, general surgery, and psychiatry. If medical students want to explore even more medical specialties such as pathology, and radiology, they can complete elective rotations. Also during medical school, students take the first parts of the USMLE (United States Medical Licensing Exam) or COMLEX (Comprehensive Osteopathic Medical Licensing Examination). In the final years of medical school, students begin applying for residency. Radiology residency is 4 years in length. First-year residents are known as interns. During residency, radiologists gain valuable experience interpreting medical images, ultrasounds, and other radiologic tests. Radiology residency is considered to be averagely competitive. After the completion of their residency, radiologists can become board-certified and consider pursuing a fellowship. Radiologists can become board-certified by passing an exam issued by The American Board of Radiology (ABR). Board certification demonstrates a physician's specialization and expertise in their field. Although board certification is not mandatory, most employers require board certification for employment. Radiologists also have the option to pursue additional training in a subspecialty of radiology. Subspecialties within radiology include pediatric radiology, breast radiology, cardiothoracic radiology, nuclear radiology, and many more. Most of these fellowships are 1-2 years in length. Many radiology residents complete multiple fellowships. After completing all of their training, radiologists must stay up-to-date with the latest research and advancements in their field. The path to becoming a radiologist opens up a world of possibilities to explore, diagnose, and contribute to the field of healthcare.

Why You Should Become a Radiologist

Work-life balance

Radiologists have a good work-life balance compared to other physicians

Technology

Radiologists have the opportunity to use lots of machinery and high-tech equipment

Puzzles

Radiologists are trained to decipher puzzling medical images to diagnose a patient

Introverted work

Radiology is known as a great specialty for people who are introverted

Radiology Trivia

1. Who discovered X-rays in 1895?
    a. Rosalind Franklin
    b. Wilhelm Roentgen
    c. Florence Nightingale
    d. Clara Barton

2. What is the main purpose of a mammogram?
    a. To detect cervical cancer
    b. To kill precancerous cells
    c. To detect breast cancer or any abnormalities in the breasts
    d. To treat breast cancer

3. When having an X-ray, why do you need to wear a lead apron?
    a. To protect from unnecessary radiation
    b. To ensure authentic X-ray results
    c. To keep the body still for the X-ray machine
    d. To protect clothing and jewelry

4. Which imaging test is commonly used to check on the development of a growing baby during pregnancy?
    a. MRIs
    b. CT scans
    c. Nuclear medicine scans
    d. Ultrasounds

All answers on next page

Radiology Trivia

1. Who discovered X-rays in 1895?

    a. Rosalind Franklin

    b. Wilhelm Roentgen

    c. Florence Nightingale

    d. Clara Barton

2. What is the main purpose of a mammogram?

    a. To detect cervical cancer

    b. To kill precancerous cells

    c. To detect breast cancer or any abnormalities in the breasts

    d. To treat breast cancer

3. When having an X-ray, why do you need to wear a lead apron?

    a. To protect from unnecessary radiation

    b. To ensure authentic X-ray results

    c. To keep the body still for the X-ray machine

    d. To protect clothing and jewelry

4. Which imaging test is commonly used to check on the development of a growing baby during pregnancy?

    a. MRIs

    b. CT scans

    c. Nuclear medicine scans

    d. Ultrasounds

Radiology Fun Facts

1. X-rays were discovered *accidentally* by Wilhelm Roentgen

2. Smoke detectors contain a small amount of radioactive material

3. The first X-ray was taken of Roentgen's wife, it was an image of her hand with her wedding ring on

4. Radium was discovered by Marie Curie in the late 19th century

5. Chest X-rays helped doctors control TB (tuberculosis)

6. Rosalind Franklin used X-ray crystallography to reveal the structure of DNA

Urology

Urology is the medical specialty that focuses on the diagnosis, treatment, and management of conditions related to the urinary and male reproductive system. The urinary system is made up of the kidneys, ureters, bladder, and urethra. The male reproductive system encompasses structures such as the testes, prostate gland, penis, and associated structures. Urologists are medical doctors who specialize in this field and are trained to provide both surgical and non-surgical treatments for a wide range of urological conditions. Urological conditions can affect individuals of all ages and genders. Urologists can treat urinary issues in men and women, but are especially experts in the male reproductive system. They can treat male infertility, prostate cancer, prostate enlargement, low testosterone levels, prostatitis, and more. Urologists also have the ability to treat UTIs (urinary tract infections), urinary incontinence (inability to control urine), hematuria (blood in urine), trouble urinating, and kidney stones. In order to treat a patient's condition a urologist must order tests. Urologists can perform rectal exams on men, and pelvic exams on women. A urinalysis is a test to determine aspects of a patient's health that requires a urine sample. Urologists may require blood tests and semen samples to diagnose and treat their patients. A urologist might also need imaging tests such as CT scans and ultrasounds to treat their patients. Urologists are trained as surgeons and can perform several complex surgeries. They can perform vasectomies (permanent male birth control), cystoscopies (examination of the lining of the bladder), lithotripsies (procedure to break down kidney stones), transurethral resections of the prostate (TURP), hydrocelectomy (removal or repair of fluid-filled sac around the testicle), varicocelectomies (treats testicular pain and increases male fertility). Urologists also perform minimally invasive procedures and robotic-assisted surgeries for a number of urological conditions. Urologists play a large role in diagnosing and treating cancers of the urinary tract, and male reproductive organs, such as bladder cancer, kidney cancer, and testicular cancer. Urologists are involved in the kidney transplantation process. They are especially involved in the surgical aspects of placing donor kidneys and connecting them to the recipient's urinary system. Urologists take great care of kidneys, and so do nephrologists. The differences and similarities between urologists and nephrologists are discussed in the chapter on Nephrology (56). The field of urology is a vital medical specialty that impacts the male reproductive system and urinary system. Urologists provide compassionate care in order to improve their patient's quality of life.

The path to becoming a urologist is filled with education, training, and a passion for urinary health and wellness. It begins with completing a bachelor's degree while fulfilling all the prerequisite courses for medical school. There is no specific major required for medical school, but majors such as biology, neuroscience, chemistry, and physics are common. Students typically take the MCAT (Medical College Admissions Test) in their third year of college or university. A high MCAT score is crucial for acceptance into medical school. A well-rounded application for medical school includes a high GPA (Grade Point Average), recommendation letters, a competitive MCAT score, research projects, and extracurricular activities. In medical school, students complete a Doctor of Medicine (M.D) or Doctor of Osteopathic Medicine (D.O) program. MDs take a more medication-focused approach to medicine while DOs take a more holistic approach to medicine. Medical school consists of classroom instruction, laboratory work, and clinical rotations in several medical specialties. Students typically rotate through specialties such as internal medicine, OB/GYN, neurosurgery, family medicine, and orthopedic surgery. If a medical student wishes to experience other specialties, they can complete elective rotations. During medical school, students take the first parts of the USMLE (United States Medical Licensing Exam) or COMLEX (Comprehensive Osteopathic Medical Licensing Exam). In the final years of medical school, students begin applying for residency. A strong residency application includes excellent letters of recommendation and clerkship scores. Urology residency is typically 5 years in length. During residency, urologists gain hands-on experience in various urological procedures and treatments, under the guidance of experienced urologists. Residents become familiar with all aspects of urology such as pediatric urology, oncology, and female urology. Also during residency, residents take the final part of the USMLE or COMLEX. After the completion of residency, urologists can consider pursuing a fellowship and becoming board certified. Fellowship isn't required, but some urologists complete fellowships in urologic oncology, pediatric urology, or male infertility. These fellowships are typically 1-2 years in length. Board certification is also not necessary, but it demonstrates a physician's level of expertise in their field. To become board certified a urologist must pass an exam by the American Board of Urology. In order to begin practicing medicine, a physician must obtain a license. After the completion of all their training, urologists must stay up-to-date with the latest advancements and techniques in their field. As urologists undergo rigorous training, they transform into experienced urologists who have the opportunity to improve patient's lives.

Urology Trivia

1. Which organ stores urine before it is released from the body?
    a. Prostate
    b. Bladder
    c. Gallbladder
    d. Kidneys

2. Which of the following is the most common type of kidney stone?
    a. Calcium oxalate
    b. Uric acid
    c. Struvite
    d. Cystine

3. What is the medical term for "bed-wetting"?
    a. Urinary incontinence
    b. Cystitis
    c. Urinary retention
    d. Urinary tract leakage

4. What is the tube that allows urine to pass outside the body?
    a. Urinary tract
    b. Testes
    c. Ureters
    d. Urethra

All answers on next page

Urology Trivia

1. Which organ stores urine before it is released from the body?

    a. Prostate

    b. Bladder

    c. Gallbladder

    d. Kidneys

2. Which of the following is the most common type of kidney stone?

    a. Calcium oxalate

    b. Uric acid

    c. Struvite

    d. Cystine

3. What is the medical term for "bed-wetting"?

    a. Urinary incontinence

    b. Cystitis

    c. Urinary retention

    d. Urinary tract leakage

4. What is the tube that allows urine to pass outside the body?

    a. Urinary tract

    b. Testes

    c. Ureters

    d. Urethra

Urology Fun Facts

1. The kidneys filter about 150 quarts of blood every day

2. The color of urine varies based on hydration levels and diet, yellow urine indicates good hydration, while dark yellow urine or light brown urine suggests dehydration

3. A healthy human bladder can hold up to 400-500 milliliters of urine, or 2 cups before it is full

4. It takes the human body 10 hours to make 2 cups of urine

5. When the bladder is empty, is it the size of a pear

6. It is normal to go to the bathroom 4-8 times a day and no more than 2 times per night

Interview with Dr. Husain

Urology

Dr. Aftab Husain M.D P.A. is a board-certified urologist who has been practicing urology since 1984. He is currently a urologist in Middlesex County, New Jersey where he owns his own practice. He completed his urology internship and residency at UMDNJ. Dr. Husain is a senior physician who has gained lots of experience throughout his career. He is a father of three, enjoys going on walks, and loves spending time with his grandchildren. Below is an interview conducted with Dr. Husain about his experience in the field of urology.

Can you share a memorable moment you've experienced in your career?

"In urology, kidney stones were a difficult problem to handle. Only surgical techniques were available to remove kidney stones, but then we came across extracorporeal shockwave lithotripsy. This technology was developed in Germany, and once this was available, the patient was placed on the machine under local anesthesia or IV sedation, and the stone was shattered by continuous shockwaves. That was huge progress and a big change in the treatment of kidney stones. After this, there was no need for open surgery to treat kidney stones, which were a major problem."

How has the field of urology evolved since you began practicing?

" A lot of changes have happened in the field of urology since I began practicing in 1984. A lot of new medications came out, there was no medicine like Flomax, which treats BPH. Two kinds of medication became available like Flomax and PROSCAR, to reduce the size of the prostate. Both of these medications made a huge difference and cut down on the number of surgeries on the prostate. And another I can remember is Viagra, there was no medication available for erectile dysfunction. Viagra, Levitra, and Cialis changed the treatment of erectile dysfunction and cut down on the number of penile prostheses and penile injections. The third thing, radical prostatectomies changed the way prostate cancer was treated. Radioactive seed implants also became available. Finally, robotic surgery changed the field of urology. There are hardly any open cases done for urologic cancer. The majority of surgeries are being done with robots."

What advice would you give someone hoping to be a urologist in the future?

"Physicians owning their own practice is rare now, most urologists have joined major groups. Medicine is changing, now we are considered providers, not doctors."

What would you say are the most rewarding aspects of being a urologist?

"The most rewarding thing is when patients come to see me and tell me that I have taken care of their family members or friends already. I have had patients tell me 'You are the best doctor in town.' That is definitely the most rewarding thing, I believe. And also the fact that I'm able to provide more time to patients and their families, which in a large medical group, would not be possible."

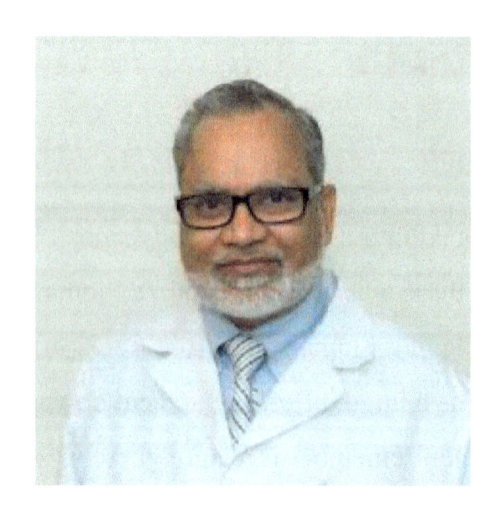

Interview with Dr. Hasan

Trauma Anesthesiology

Dr. Zain Hasan D.O. is an experienced, board-certified trauma anesthesiologist. He currently practices in Los Angeles, California. He is an expert in regional anesthesia and nerve blocks. Dr. Hasan is also a father of 1 and content creator. He enjoys spending time on social media, fitness, and working out. Below is an interview conducted with Dr. Hasan about his experience in the field of trauma anesthesiology.

What inspired you to specialize in trauma anesthesiology?

"It was a field that I think connected most with my interests, it has realms of both surgery and medicine, which is hard to find. In trauma anesthesiology, you cover every kind of emergency out there. That to me, made me feel like I would make an impact in people's lives without pursuing surgery itself. It genuinely makes an impact."

Can you describe your typical workday as an anesthesiologist?

"My day usually starts at 5:00 o'clock, and I get to the hospital at about 6:30. I see my patients prepare for their surgery, and figure out a plan. Depending on if I'm supervising, or if I'm doing my own cases, either I see 1 patient or 3 patients in the morning. Then whatever surgeries are scheduled I do those. If there are any emergencies, like traumas, those come in and I do those. By the evening, I'm usually done by 4 or 5 o'clock. Occasionally, once a week I take a call, usually overnight."

What advice would you give to med students or residents interested in pursuing anesthesiology?

"It's become a lot more competitive in the last couple of years since COVID-19. It is a lot more shift-work sort of, there's a lot less calls and those kinds of things. But it's definitely become a lot more competitive, so you have to work hard and do well on your boards. Do well on your sub-internships, make friends with the attendings who are involved in the selection process, and go from there!"

What are the most critical skills or qualities that a successful anesthesiologist should have?

"That's a good question, they need to be able to work under pressure in time-constrained situations. You're dealing with life and death, and you have maybe 90 seconds to make the right decision to save someone's life during surgery, whether it's when they're going to sleep, waking up, or in the middle of surgery. You have to be able to function under short bursts of high stress, and there's a lot of downtime too. Overall, you just have to be able to deal with pressure."

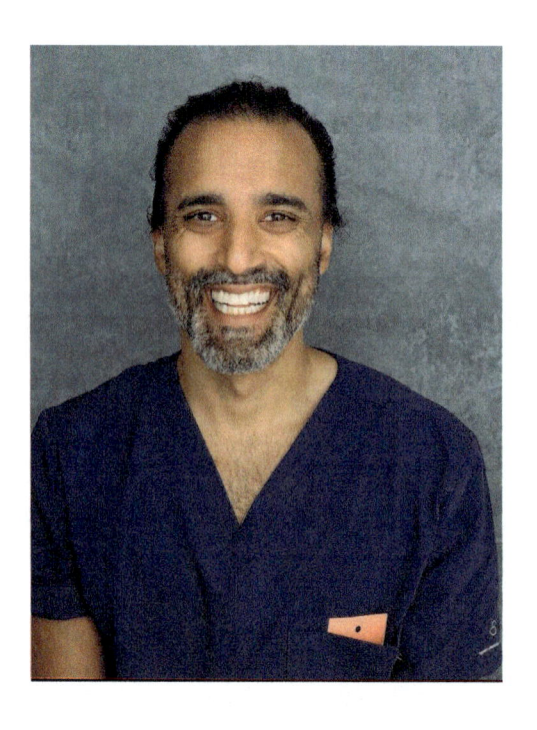

Author's Note

As I reflect on the journey that led to the creation of *Decoding Medical Careers: A Teenage Guide to Medical Specialties,* I realize that I couldn't be more thrilled to share it with you. Firstly, I extend my gratitude to my parents whose encouragement has been my motivation throughout this journey. I especially thank them for never getting annoyed by the endless hours I spoke about this book. I also extend thanks towards my grandfather, Dr. Husain who generously shared his insights and experiences through interviews. I thank Fizza Zaidi who assisted me with getting the most out of these interviews. I especially thank Dr. Hasan whose perspectives added tremendous amounts of depth to the pages of this book, no matter how many times I reached out to him. To my readers, I began this writing journey with hopes of inspiring teenagers like me to delve into the world of medical specialties. I encourage readers to consider the endless possibilities of each medical career. Each field holds its own challenges and rewards, and they are waiting to be explored. Writing this book has been a transformative experience for me as well. The research, interviews, and late nights discovering more about each specialty has expanded my understanding of the medical field. I've gained valuable information about medicine that I hope to share with others. One of my goals in crafting this book was to shed light on the many careers and specialties in medicine. It is my hope that readers find inspiration within these pages, allowing them to consider pursuing a career in medicine. As you read *Decoding Medical Careers: A Teenage Guide to Medical Specialties,* remember that the medical world is large and constantly evolving. Let the stories of medical professionals and the detailed descriptions of each specialty inspire you. Thanks for decoding all 20 medical specialties with me!

Printed in Dunstable, United Kingdom